The WITH or WITHOUT {MEAT} Cookbook

The Flexible Approach to Flavorful Diabetes Cooking

Jackie Newgent, RDN, CDN

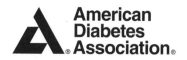

American Diabetes Association

Director, Book Publishing, Abe Ogden; *Managing Editor,* Greg Guthrie; *Acquisitions Editor,* Victor Van Beuren; *Production Manager and Composition,* Melissa Sprott; *Cover Design,* pixiedesign, llc; *Photographer,* Cameron Whitman Photography; *Printer:* Marquis Imprimeur.

Printed in Canada

1 3 5 7 9 10 8 6 4 2

The suggestions and information contained in this publication are generally consistent with the *Clinical Practice Recommendations* and other policies of the American Diabetes Association, but they do not represent the policy or position of the Association or any of its boards or committees. Reasonable steps have been taken to ensure the accuracy of the information presented. However, the American Diabetes Association cannot ensure the safety or efficacy of any product or service described in this publication. Individuals are advised to consult a physician or other appropriate health care professional before undertaking any diet or exercise program or taking any medication referred to in this publication. Professionals must use and apply their own professional judgment, experience, and training and should not rely solely on the information contained in this publication before prescribing any diet, exercise, or medication. The American Diabetes Association—its officers, directors, employees, volunteers, and members—assumes no responsibility or liability for personal or other injury, loss, or damage that may result from the suggestions or information in this publication.

♾ The paper in this publication meets the requirements of the ANSI Standard Z39.48-1992 (permanence of paper).

ADA titles may be purchased for business or promotional use or for special sales. To purchase more than 50 copies of this book at a discount, or for custom editions of this book with your logo, contact the American Diabetes Association at the address below, at booksales@diabetes.org, or by calling 703-299-2046.

American Diabetes Association
1701 North Beauregard Street
Alexandria, Virginia 22311

Front cover image: Caprese Avocado "Cheeseburger," p. 154–155.
Back cover images: Roasted Vegetable Wrap, p. 136; Peppercorn Pistachio Caesar-Style Salad, p. 36.

DOI: 10.2337/9781580405164

Library of Congress Cataloging-in-Publication Data

Newgent, Jackie.
  The with or without meat cookbook / Jackie Newgent.
      pages cm
  Summary: "This book will provide the reader with healthy recipes, whether cooking with meat or a vegetarian-based meal"-- Provided by publisher.
  Includes bibliographical references and index.
  ISBN 978-1-58040-516-4 (paperback : alkaline paper) 1. Vegetarian cooking. 2. Meat. 3. Diabetes--Diet therapy--Recipes. I. American Diabetes Association. II. Title.
  TX837.N514 2014
  641.5'636--dc23
                              2013030965

In memory of my mother, Jean (Rafool) Newgent

Table of Contents

Acknowledgments

I'm so appreciative of the many people who have helped make this cookbook a reality.

A special thank you to my father, Richard Newgent, for inspiring me to make a difference in the eating habits and health of people with diabetes.

To my sister, Rebecca. Thank you for your help and insight while double-testing some of the book's recipes.

To Maureen Varnon, my business colleague. Thank you for your professional and media guidance.

To Beth Shepard, my agent. Thank you for your years of support.

To Stephanie Smith and Lea Loveland, my wonderful interns. Thank you both for your culinary nutrition enthusiasm and creative spirits.

To Cameron Whitman and Danielle Esposti, the photography team for *The With or Without Meat Cookbook*. Thank you for making my recipes jump off the page.

To the editors and behind-the-scenes expertise at the American Diabetes Association, including Abe Ogden, Greg Guthrie, Victor Van Beuren, and Melissa Sprott. You've been a delight to work with. Thank you everyone!

Introduction

The *With or Without Meat Cookbook* makes it simple for everyone to savor the tastes and enjoy the health benefits of a plant-centered eating plan. The recipes are ideal for people with or at risk for diabetes, but are helpful for anyone trying to manage a healthy weight. The most intriguing feature of this cookbook, however, is that whether you're a plant lover or a meat eater, the dishes can be customized to your preferences. Pair this feature with the deliciousness of the recipes, and you've got a cookbook fit for anyone's taste buds!

Now there's no more fixing two different meals to try to please all. Since the recipes are flexible, you can make one recipe even if you're cooking for someone who eats meat and someone who does not. You can also change it up and prepare a recipe with meat one day and without meat another day. The popular name for this type of eating plan is flexitarianism. A flexitarian is someone who eats plant-based meals and may occasionally eat poultry, fish, or meat. This is considered by nutrition experts, including myself, to be a desirable and wholesome approach to eating.

NUTRITIONAL HIGHLIGHTS

Creatively prepared veggies and whole grains take center stage in *The With or Without Meat Cookbook*. All recipes use real ingredients, and they all meet the following diabetes-friendly nutritional criteria per serving.

Maximum of:

♦ 400 calories
♦ 45g total carbohydrate (with an emphasis on whole grains); most recipes are 30g total carbohydrate or less
♦ 0g trans fat and very low saturated fat
♦ 600mg sodium (meals or main dishes); 480mg sodium (all other recipes)

1

"WITH POULTRY, FISH, OR MEAT"

Here are the specifics for what makes *The With or Without Meat Cookbook* so unique. Each of the 125 diabetes-friendly recipes is vegetarian but includes a non-vegetarian recipe option labeled "With Poultry, Fish, or Meat" so that every single recipe can be prepared two ways: for both veggie fans and meat lovers. This flexitarian-style "add-on" is just like it sounds; you'll only need to take the time and energy to prepare one full recipe. The "add-on" is an individual ingredient or extra-simple recipe that's incorporated into as much of the original plant-based recipe as desired.

For instance, instead of making two entirely different recipes, such as a veggie burrito and a meaty burrito, one recipe for a Stewed Green Burrito (page 156) is provided. The "With Poultry, Fish, or Meat" option of grilled strips of pork tenderloin can be incorporated into one or more servings of the plant-centered recipe. (See "How to Use this Flexible Cookbook," below.) The bottom line: these recipes are perfect for couples or families that have both vegetarians and non-vegetarians dining together.

HOW TO USE THIS FLEXIBLE COOKBOOK

1. FOR VEGETARIANS AND PLANT-BASED EATERS

Use the main recipes as written. If you're preparing food for yourself and one or more non-vegetarians, use the "With Poultry, Fish, or Meat" option listed as "One serving." Multiply this single serving, if needed. For vegans, note that more than half of the recipes fit your eating style. See the vegan recipe index (page 259–260).

2. FOR NON-VEGETARIANS

If you eat poultry, fish, or meat, you can use the main recipes without meat or you can use the "With Poultry, Fish, or Meat" option listed as "Full recipe." Gradually wean yourself off of the "With Poultry, Fish, or Meat" options to enjoy the main recipes within a plant-based diet.

Regardless of which way you choose to prepare the recipes, know that they're all plant-centered dishes. You won't find a steak bigger than your plate in this book! The elective animal products are included in responsible, healthful, and desirable ways. When you do decide on the "With Poultry, Fish, or Meat" selection, it'll be a petite piece that's used more like a delightful addition—like a sidekick, not the star of the show. For many, this may be a new way of appreciating meat, poultry, and fish. It'll add another taste element to the main meatless recipes, but the recipes are full-flavored either way.

When you take the option, each recipe provides up to 3 ounces poultry, fish, or meat per serving. In many cases, it may be just 1/2 ounce. It takes time to adapt to using meat as a minor ingredient, but you will adjust. Actually, when meat is served this way, you'll be able to truly appreciate and want to savor every bite. What's more, you'll be able to enjoy some decadent selections since the amount of meat is kept to just a little, not a lot. Go with the eco-friendliest picks when possible to feel good about what you're savoring, too. (See "Go Eco," below.) Finally, don't worry about buying poultry, fish, or meat in these petite portions; you can almost always buy larger portions, use what you need, and freeze the rest.

GO ECO

If you decide to prepare the "With Poultry, Fish, or Meat" options, I recommend choosing organic poultry, sustainable fish and shellfish, and organic, grass-fed meat when possible. (For some of my favorite picks, see "Product Recommendations" pages 243–246.) I developed and tested the recipes with these choices in mind. Look for the USDA Certified Organic seal. These "clean" options are better for your health and the planet. Among the many benefits: organic poultry and meat is antibiotic-free and raised on a diet that's free of genetically modified organisms (GMOs). Grass-fed meat is generally leaner and more nutrient rich than its grain-fed counterpart. Products like organic deli meat or organic bacon won't have the addition of potentially cancer-causing preservatives, like nitrites or nitrates, and tend to be lower in sodium overall. And sustainable, eco-friendly seafood won't carry high levels of harmful toxins, like polychlorinated biphenyls (PCBs) and mercury. Go to seafoodwatch.org for an updated list of the eco-best and healthiest fish and shellfish selections.

The "With Poultry, Fish, or Meat" versions can usually be served just like the original version of the recipe…a side dish remains a side dish, for example. However, these flexitarian recipe options occasionally turn a non-entrée recipe into an entrée. In these cases, simply plan the rest of your meal accordingly. Use the provided nutrition information as a guide to planning your entire meal. You'll see nutrition analysis labeled as "without," which corresponds to each serving of the main vegetarian recipe, and as "with," which corresponds to each serving of the poultry, fish, or meat version. By the way, the poultry, fish, and meat recipe versions meet the diabetes-friendly nutrition criteria established for the main meat-free recipes, too.

RECIPE FEATURES

Along with the nutrition criteria, The With or Without Meat Cookbook has three key recipe features:

1. Fresh & Flavorful
   - Taste is the primary focus; high-quality ingredients are recommended
   - The food philosophy is "fresh is best"; plenty of fresh vegetables and herbs are included
   - All-natural whole ingredients are the focus; absolutely nothing is artificial

2. Nutrient Rich
   - Veggies are part of nearly every recipe; whole grains are used in place of refined grains
   - Highly processed ingredients aren't advised
   - For the flexitarian option, organic poultry/meat and sustainable fish are recommended

3. Simple
   - Recipes rely mainly on readily available ingredients that you know and love
   - Instructions are easy to follow and do not require complicated techniques
   - "Natural" convenience foods, like prepackaged salad greens or organic canned beans, help save time

MEDITERRANEAN DIET

This cookbook isn't just considered plant-centered or flexitarian. It's developed mainly on the principles of a Mediterranean-style diet. So if you want to be specific, *The With or Without Meat Cookbook* follows a Mediterranean-style flexitarian approach.

Overall, the Mediterranean diet is considered to be one of the most nutritious eating styles. Research shows it can reduce the risk of heart disease as well as play a beneficial role in the prevention of some major chronic diseases.

Here's what you'll find in the Mediterranean diet that you'll also find in *The With or Without Meat Cookbook*:

- ◆ Plant-based recipes, including whole grains, vegetables, fruits, beans, nuts, and seeds
- ◆ Emphasis on fresh foods
- ◆ Herbs and spices used liberally
- ◆ Olive oil as one of the preferred cooking fats
- ◆ Moderate portions of eggs, cheese, and yogurt
- ◆ Small amounts of meat—and only as an option

It's important to know that a Mediterranean-style eating plan is beyond just a diet. In order to reap more of its benefits, you'll want to sit down and fully enjoy your meals with others. That also means no electronic devices at the table! Plenty of exercise is important, too, of course.

What's more, along with the Mediterranean-style flexitarian approach that I use for the recipes, you'll see some global influences to keep the dishes exciting. Also, since my heritage is half Lebanese, I've sprinkled in some of my personal cultural influences to make this cookbook still more enticing, while sharing the food that I find brings much pleasure.

PLANT-BASED CONSIDERATIONS

When you move veggies and whole grains to the center of the plate, it can mean less protein on the plate. Getting ample protein on a vegetarian or flexitarian eating plan may become problematic if your meals are not properly planned. Pay special attention to nutrition information provided on food labels and recipes. Choose "real" foods first. And try some of these simple suggestions to assure your plant-rich diet is also protein rich:

◆ **Go big on beans.** Soybeans are a particularly good source of protein. You can enjoy any of the many forms including tofu, baked ready-to-eat tofu, canned soybeans, and edamame. Choose certified organic soybean products to assure they're not genetically modified—otherwise known as GMO-free. Try an array of beans as sides and starters, including hummus and various bean dips.

◆ **Top with nuts.** Almonds, pistachios, and peanuts are versatile culinary nuts, and all provide significant protein. Sprinkle these onto veggie entrées and sides for added crunch and eye appeal.

◆ **Enjoy a heaping spoonful of hemp.** You can buy it as raw shelled seeds, sometimes called hemp hearts. A 3-tablespoon serving of the seeds provides 10 grams of protein. Stir into baked-good batters or sprinkle onto salads. Or do what I do and just eat a big spoonful—straight from the spoon, if you like.

◆ **Pick vegetarian "substitutes" wisely.** Some meatless items that are developed to replace meat can be overly processed and taste fake. Luckily, better tasting, more minimally processed options are now showing up on store shelves. Read ingredient lists and choose foods where the list reads rather like a recipe, not a science experiment.

◆ **Try lacto-ovo vegetarianism.** Eggs (especially the egg whites) and dairy foods (notably Greek yogurt) are excellent sources of high-quality protein. Consider keeping these foods in a vegetarian eating plan.

◆ **Rethink your sides.** Poultry, fish, and meat don't need to be main dishes. They can make succulent side dishes and meal accents if you're following a flexitarian eating plan.

When preparing both vegetarian and non-vegetarian meals, "cross-contamination" needs to be considered. This term is often used to discuss food safety. You don't want ready-to-eat foods and raw meat, poultry, or fish to come into contact. In the case of a plant-based diet, however, the term refers to any meat, poultry, or fish coming into contact with any plant-based foods during storing, cooking, serving, or dining. Avoiding this type of "cross-contamination" is an absolute "rule" for true vegetarians. Always make sure to separate the meat, poultry, or fish dish from the vegetarian-friendly food. Try baking it in a separate pan or mixing it in a separate bowl with a separate spoon. When grilling, plan to grill meat, poultry, or fish next to or preferably after the vegetarian item, not before. When serving nearly identical dishes, consider garnishing the meaty dish differently than the meatless dish so everyone can easily differentiate them.

TOP REASONS TO FOLLOW A PLANT-BASED EATING APPROACH

It's clear that eating a plant-rich diet is good for you. Research finds that people who follow plant-based eating plans are generally slimmer, healthier, and tend to have lower risks of diabetes, cardiovascular disease, and cancer than do people who eat a meat-laden diet. Here's more motivation to keep following this eating style for good:

- ◆ Great taste
- ◆ Bigger portions
- ◆ Increased satiety
- ◆ Fewer calories
- ◆ More nutrients
- ◆ Visual appeal
- ◆ Lower cost
- ◆ Animal welfare
- ◆ Environmentally friendly

TOP VEGGIE TIPS

Are you already regularly eating plenty of veggies? Congratulations! If not, I have some clever tips to help you do so. You know by now that I suggest following a plant-centered approach to eating, but that doesn't mean simply placing a veggie side dish onto the center of your plate and calling it an entrée. It does mean, however, serving vegetables in a manner that looks and satisfies like a main dish.

How to Make Vegetables the Star of Your Plate

♦ **Make it a "steak"!** Cut an entire head of cauliflower into thick slices. Do the same with eggplant or an oversized vegetable of choice. Roast or grill them and dress them up, too! See Roasted Cauliflower Florentine (page 20) and Grilled Eggplant Steak (page 170).

♦ **Celebrate mushrooms' meatiness.** Mushrooms provide a savory or "meaty" taste called "umami." Sauté sliced mushrooms and stuff into sandwiches in place of beef, lamb, pork, or veal. You can also grill a large portabella mushroom and serve as a smoky burger patty. Make Maitake Gyro (page 140) and Caprese Avocado "Cheeseburger" (page 154).

♦ **Try tofu transformations.** Tofu is made from soybeans so it counts as a veggie. Scramble it just like eggs and add a pinch of turmeric to provide a natural yellow hue. Or slice, marinate, and grill it, and savor any way you like. Enjoy Sunrise Scrambled Squash and Poblano Tacos (page 22) and Hot Madras Curried Tofu Salad (page 88).

♦ **Make grains greater.** Marry seasonal veggies with quinoa or whole-wheat couscous and give it the special treatment by molding it. Or top a petite whole-grain pasta portion generously with veggies, like several roasted asparagus spears packed together in alternating fashion to create a grand-appearing dish. Pick Mint Pesto Couscous and Peas (page 182) and Roasted Asparagus Parmigiana with Pasta (page 190).

♦ **Double up.** Toss noodles with an equal or greater amount of seasonal veggies to double the portion size without doubling the calories. Try Orecchiette and Kale with Pecorino Romano (page 194) and Veggie Chow Fun (page 202).

♦ **Prepare like pasta.** Cut zucchini or yellow summer squash into long strips using a vegetable peeler or, if you have one, a mandoline. Then, prepare them as if they're fettuccine, linguine, or Asian-style noodles. Use roasted spaghetti squash just like spaghetti, too. Check out Satay Zucchini Noodles (page 166) and Spaghetti Squash a Cacio e Pepe (page 230).

♦ **Stack it or stick it.** Go for a wow effect or a playful touch. Build a colorful stack of prepared seasonal vegetables, and serve attractively on a ladleful of sauce. Or, simply skewer several veggies along with tofu, and grill. Show these off: Garnet Yam Stack (page 180) and Tzatziki Tofu and Vegetable Kebabs (page 174).

20 Easiest Tips Ever for Boosting Veggies

1. Make half your plate or bowl nonstarchy veggies.
2. Choose vegetables that you love.
3. Go heavy on fresh herbs.
4. Pick packaged salads and pre-prepped veggies.
5. Keep colorful crudités in plain sight in the fridge.
6. Serve creamy hummus as a veggie dip or condiment.
7. Savor grape tomatoes as an anytime snack.
8. Swap portabella mushrooms for meat.
9. Make sandwiches top heavy with crisp veggies.
10. Enjoy edamame as a versatile appetizer.
11. Cut and bake a veggie of choice to serve like fries.
12. Drink your veggies in place of soda.
13. Have a quick-fix stash of frozen vegetables.
14. Stock up on canned beans for protein in a pinch.
15. Munch on crunchy freeze-dried vegetables on the go.
16. Grab a slice of pizza…veggie pizza.
17. Order vegetarian when dining out.
18. Swing by the salad bar instead of the fast food drive-thru.
19. Hit the farmers' market every weekend.
20. Celebrate "Meatless Mondays"—and other days of the week.

Meat-Free Meals

To transform a recipe into a meal, these simple and well-planned vegetarian menu ideas will give you a delicious starting point. Pick them based on seasonality of produce, when possible. Every breakfast, lunch, and dinner serving provides about 400 calories and no more than 45g total carbohydrates, so each meal should easily fit into your eating plan.

BREAKFASTS

EGG WHITE PANINI PLATE
Portabella, Rosemary Egg White, and Greens Panini (page 26)
1 medium orange
1/4 Hass avocado, sliced
Per serving: 380 calories (44g total carbohydrate)

SUMMERTIME BREAKFAST TACOS
Sunrise Scrambled Squash and Poblano Tacos (page 22)
1 medium peach
Per serving: 370 calories (45g total carbohydrate)

REINVENTED EGG-FREE FLORENTINE
Roasted Cauliflower Florentine (page 20)
25 almonds
6 unsulphured dried apricot halves
Per serving: 380 calories (40g total carbohydrate)

ANYTIME EGGS AND TOAST
Herbed 'Shroom and Egg Scramble (page 14)
1 slice whole-grain toast with 1 tablespoon almond butter and
        2 teaspoons 100% fruit spread
1 small apple
Per serving: 390 calories (45g total carbohydrate)

LUNCHES

CURRY CHICK'N SALAD PLATTER
Hot Madras Curried Tofu Salad (page 88)
1 ounce small whole-grain crackers
2/3 cup blackberries or blueberries
22 dry-roasted pistachios
Per serving: 400 calories (43g total carbohydrate)

MEDITERRANEAN SALAD WITH HUMMUS
Fresh Mint and Baby Spinach Salad with Grapes (page 72)
1/2 whole-grain pita
1/3 cup hummus drizzled with 1 teaspoon extra-virgin olive oil
Per serving: 380 calories (45g total carbohydrate)

CIABATTA, CHEESE, AND CHERRIES
Mozzarella, Arugula, and Plum Ciabatta (page 148)
1 cup low-fat (1%), low-sodium cottage cheese
10 cherries
Per serving: 410 calories (45g total carbohydrate)

IT'S A WRAP
Chimichurri Hummus and Cauliflower Wrap (page 138)
1 1/2 tablespoons unsalted sunflower seeds
Per serving: 400 calories (41g total carbohydrate)

DINNERS

GRILL OUT FOR GUESTS

Grilled Spring Asparagus Salad (page 70)
Garnet Yam Stack (page 180)
1 tablespoon toasted pine nuts, for garnishing
Per serving: 390 calories (36g total carbohydrate)

SPICY QUESADILLA DINNER

Black Bean and Sweet Potato Quesadilla (page 158)
    with 2 tablespoons guacamole of choice (page 159)
1 cup sautéed spinach or other leafy greens
    with 1 teaspoon extra-virgin olive oil and hot pepper flakes to taste
Per serving: 380 calories (43g total carbohydrate)

GRECIAN KEBABS ON QUINOA

Tzatziki Tofu and Vegetable Kebabs (page 174)
3/4 cup steamed quinoa with 1 tablespoon toasted sliced almonds,
    1 teaspoon extra-virgin olive oil, fresh mint to taste, and a lemon wedge
Per serving: 400 calories (42g total carbohydrate)

SAVORY TRIO

Saucy Mushrooms (page 216)
Sticky Thai Quinoa (page 232)
Szechuan Edamame (page 237)
Per serving: 390 calories (44g total carbohydrate)

CHAPTER 1

breakfast and brunch

Herbed 'Shroom and Egg Scramble

Makes 4 servings: 1/2 cup each

2 large organic eggs

4 large organic egg whites or 1/2 cup pasteurized 100% egg whites

2 tablespoons plain unsweetened almond milk or other plant-based milk

1/4 teaspoon freshly ground black pepper, or to taste

1/8 teaspoon sea salt, or to taste

1/8 teaspoon ground turmeric

1 1/2 teaspoons canola or grapeseed oil

1 (8-ounce) package fresh crimini mushrooms, very thinly sliced

2 scallions, thinly sliced with green and white parts separated

1 teaspoon chopped fresh rosemary

1/4 cup shredded French Raclette or aged Swiss cheese (1 ounce)

If you're a fan of mushrooms, these scrambled eggs are made for your taste buds. The mushrooms add an earthy savoriness that makes this breakfast entrée special. The turmeric imparts a rich yellow hue, which makes it extra unique, and it'll seem like you've used more yolks than you have. Enjoy this full-flavored favorite along with whole-grain toast and roasted tomato halves.

1. Whisk together the eggs, egg whites, almond milk, pepper, salt, and turmeric in a small bowl. Set aside.

2. Heat the oil in a large, nonstick skillet over medium heat. Add the mushrooms, white part of the scallions, and the rosemary. Sauté until the mushrooms are fully wilted, about 7 minutes. Stir in the green part of the scallions.

3. Pour in the egg mixture and cook while scrambling until the eggs are no longer runny, about 4 minutes. Stir in the cheese.

4. Transfer the egg mixture to a platter or individual plates, and serve.

{ WITH POULTRY, FISH, OR MEAT }

One serving: Dice 1 ounce thick-sliced lean uncured Virginia ham. Heat in a separate skillet over medium heat until hot, about 2 minutes. Stir 1/2 cup of the egg mixture into the ham after stirring in the cheese in step 3.

Full recipe: Dice 4 ounces thick-sliced lean uncured Virginia ham. Add to the skillet along with the green part of the scallions in step 2.

without

Exchanges/Food Choices: 1 Vegetable, 1 Lean Meat, 1 Fat
120 calories, 60 calories from fat, 7g total fat, 2.5g saturated fat, 0g trans fat,
100mg cholesterol, 200mg sodium,
380mg potassium, 4g total carbohydrate,
1g dietary fiber, 2g sugars, 10g protein,
168mg phosphorus

with

Exchanges/Food Choices: 1 Vegetable, 2 Lean Meat, 1 Fat
150 calories, 60 calories from fat, 7g total fat, 2.5g saturated fat, 0g trans fat,
120mg cholesterol, 370mg sodium,
460mg potassium, 4g total carbohydrate,
1g dietary fiber, 2g sugars, 17g protein,
220mg phosphorus

Nonstick Skillets

I frequently suggest the use of nonstick skillets in recipes. It allows for just the right amount of oil or other cooking fat to be added to a recipe—and sometimes none at all. However, I only suggest using nonstick skillets and other pans that are PFOA-free. In laboratory animals, PFOA, or perfluorooctanoic acid, has caused adverse developmental effects and may be carcinogenic. So, the safest bet for everyone is to steer clear of this chemical. Contact the manufacturer of your nonstick cookware to find out if it's free of PFOA. Alternatively, use cast-iron skillets. When they are well seasoned, they provide an excellent stick-resistant cooking surface.

Scrambled Huevos Rancheros Bowl

2 large organic eggs

5 large organic egg whites or 2/3 cup pasteurized 100% egg whites

2 tablespoons plain unsweetened almond milk or other plant-based milk

1 small jalapeño pepper, without seeds, minced

1/2 teaspoon finely chopped fresh oregano leaves

1/4 teaspoon sea salt, or to taste

1/8 teaspoon ground turmeric

1 1/2 teaspoons canola or unrefined peanut oil

2 tomatillos, husks removed and rinsed, finely diced

1 cup cooked or drained canned pinto beans, patted dry

8 unsalted red or blue corn tortilla chips, whole or broken

1/2 Hass avocado, peeled, pitted, and diced

1/4 cup mild or medium tomatillo salsa (salsa verde)

2 tablespoons sour cream

2 tablespoon fresh cilantro leaves

For a zesty and rápido start to your day, gather and pre-prep most of the ingredients the night before you plan to make this. It's kind of like breakfast tacos, but all scrambled up into a delicious concoction that's meant to be savored one luscious forkful at a time. The result is a bowl of flavor, fun, and filling satisfaction. To round out the meal with extra deliciousness, serve with slices of the remaining avocado half on the side along with a cup of fresh seasonal fruit.

1. Whisk together the eggs, egg whites, almond milk, jalapeño, oregano, salt, and turmeric in a medium bowl.

2. Heat the oil in a large, nonstick skillet over medium heat. Add the egg mixture and tomatillos and cook while scrambling until the eggs are no longer runny, about 5 minutes. Stir in the beans and chips and cook for 30 seconds. Adjust seasoning.

3. Transfer the egg mixture to individual bowls. Top with the avocado and salsa. Dollop with the sour cream, sprinkle with the cilantro leaves, and serve.

{ WITH POULTRY, FISH, OR MEAT }

One serving: Slice a 1-ounce portion of a precooked, spicy poultry sausage link into thin "coins." Cook in a small, nonstick skillet over medium heat until fully heated through. Stir in 3/4 cup (one serving without toppings) egg mixture at the end of step 2. Serve without the sour cream.

Full recipe: Slice 4 ounces precooked, spicy poultry sausage links into thin "coins." Add to the hot oil in step 2 and cook until fully heated through. Then pour in the egg mixture. Serve without the sour cream.

without
Exchanges/Food Choices: 1 Starch,
1 Vegetable, 1 Medium-Fat Meat, 1 Fat
200 calories, 80 calories from fat, 9g total fat,
2g saturated fat, 0g trans fat,
100mg cholesterol, 390mg sodium,
420mg potassium, 16g total carbohydrate,
6g dietary fiber, 3g sugars, 12g protein,
140mg phosphorus

with
Exchanges/Food Choices: 1 Starch,
1 Vegetable, 1 Medium-Fat Meat, 1 1/2 Fat
230 calories, 100 calories from fat, 11g total
fat, 2.5g saturated fat, 0g trans fat,
115mg cholesterol, 590mg sodium,
480mg potassium, 17g total carbohydrate,
6g dietary fiber, 3g sugars, 16g protein,
190mg phosphorus

Dry Beans

Canned beans are super convenient. When using them, I suggest selecting an organic variety, so all that's in the can are beans, water, and sometimes salt or sea salt. However, if you prefer to use dried beans, here's how to prepare them: Rinse 1 pound beans well and discard any stones. Add the beans and 10–12 cups water to a large pot or bowl. Refrigerate overnight or about 8 hours. Drain, rinse the beans, and return the beans to the large pot. Cover the beans with water, about 3 inches above bean level (add more water during cooking, if necessary). Bring to a boil. Then, reduce the heat to low and simmer uncovered, stirring occasionally, until tender, about 1 hour and 15 minutes (cooking time may vary). Drain beans and use in recipe, or add the beans to ice cold water until just cool, drain well, and freeze in 1- or 1 1/2-cup packages. Yields about 5 cups cooked beans.

Baby Spinach and Feta Frittata

Makes 1 serving: 1 frittata

1 1/2 teaspoons extra-virgin olive oil

1 scallion, green and white parts, minced

3 cups packed fresh baby spinach (3 ounces)

1 teaspoon fresh lemon juice

1/8 teaspoon freshly grated or ground nutmeg

1/8 teaspoon dried hot pepper flakes

1 tablespoon crumbled feta cheese

5 large organic egg whites or 2/3 cup pasteurized 100% egg whites

1/8 teaspoon freshly ground black pepper, or to taste

without
Exchanges/Food Choices: 1 1/2 Vegetable, 2 Lean Meat, 1 1/2 Fat
210 calories, 80 calories from fat,
9g total fat, 2.5g saturated fat, 0g trans fat,
10mg cholesterol, 520mg sodium,
300mg potassium, 13g total carbohydrate,
5g dietary fiber, 1g sugars, 21g protein,
60mg phosphorus

with
Exchanges/Food Choices: 1 1/2 Vegetable, 5 Lean Meat, 1 1/2 Fat
340 calories, 110 calories from fat,
12g total fat, 3.3g saturated fat, 0g trans fat,
75mg cholesterol, 570mg sodium,
500mg potassium, 13g total carbohydrate,
5g dietary fiber, 1g sugars, 46g protein,
240mg phosphorus

For the no-yolk eater, here's a brilliant, Grecian-inspired breakfast (or lunch or dinner) entrée for one. It's loaded with spinach, so the frittata fills up your entire plate! The right amount of feta creates tangy pops of flavor to wake up your palate. Be sure to crumble it as finely as possible so a little bit gets into every bite. What's more, this frittata is packed with protein, so it'll provide plenty of satiation. Pair it with fresh or toasted whole-grain pita to make it a meal.

1. Heat the oil in a large, nonstick skillet over medium heat. Add the scallion and spinach, and cook while tossing with tongs until the spinach is just wilted, about 2 1/2 minutes. Add the lemon juice, nutmeg, and hot pepper flakes, and stir to combine.

2. Evenly sprinkle with the feta cheese and add the egg whites and black pepper, gently shaking the skillet to assure the egg whites are evenly distributed. Cover and cook until the egg whites are cooked through, about 4 minutes. Adjust seasoning.

3. Loosen the frittata from the skillet using a spatula, carefully slide or flip out onto a plate, and serve.

{ WITH POULTRY, FISH, OR MEAT }

For one serving (full recipe): Season 1/2 cup chopped roasted, grilled, or poached chicken breast meat with 1/8 teaspoon ground cinnamon. (Hint: Leftovers work great!) Then sprinkle into the skillet along with the feta cheese in step 2.

Savory Mediterranean Oats

Makes 1 serving: 1 rounded cup

When it's all about cooking just for you, treat yourself to this clever morning main dish designed for one. Think of it like a creamy risotto, but with oats as the grain of choice. The goat cheese and basil provide an unforgettable finishing touch. After discovering this savory way to prepare oatmeal, you might not want to go back to a sweetened bowl of it again.

1. Bring the broth, sun-dried tomatoes, salt, and pepper to a boil in a small saucepan.

2. Stir in the oats and chives, and reduce heat to medium. Stir, until the oats are fully cooked, about 5 minutes. Remove from the heat and stir in the yogurt. Adjust seasoning.

3. Transfer to a bowl, sprinkle with the basil and goat cheese, and serve.

{ WITH POULTRY, FISH, OR MEAT }

For one serving (full recipe): Do not add salt to the recipe. Instead of sprinkling with goat cheese in step 3, place 1/2 ounce thinly sliced speck (dry-cured smoked Italian ham) or prosciutto on top of the grits like it's a rose.

1 cup low-sodium vegetable broth

4 large sun-dried tomato halves, not oil-packed, thinly sliced (do not rehydrate)

Pinch sea salt, or to taste

1/8 teaspoon freshly ground black pepper, or to taste

1/2 cup old-fashioned rolled oats

1 tablespoon minced fresh chives

3 tablespoons plain fat-free Greek yogurt

1 tablespoon thinly sliced fresh basil

1 tablespoon crumbled soft goat cheese

without
Exchanges/Food Choices: 2 Starch, 1 Vegetable, 1/2 Fat
240 calories, 50 calories from fat, 5g total fat, 2g saturated fat, 0g trans fat, 5mg cholesterol, 360mg sodium, 300mg potassium, 37g total carbohydrate, 6g dietary fiber, 8g sugars, 12g protein, 60mg phosphorus

with
Exchanges/Food Choices: 2 Starch, 1 Vegetable, 1 Fat
240 calories, 45 calories from fat, 5g total fat, 1g saturated fat, 0g trans fat, 10mg cholesterol, 560mg sodium, 370mg potassium, 37g total carbohydrate, 6g dietary fiber, 8g sugars, 14g protein, 80mg phosphorus

Roasted Cauliflower Florentine

Makes 4 servings: 1 topped cauliflower slice each

Need to impress? Here's a beauty of a breakfast. This surprisingly low-calorie, special-occasion version of eggs Florentine, served on caramelized cauliflower in place of English muffin, topped with oozy roasted tomato instead of poached egg, and ladled with a delicious and velvety sauce instead of über-rich hollandaise, meets that challenge scrumptiously and stunningly.

4 (1-inch thick) whole slices from a large head cauliflower* (about 6.5 ounces per slice)

2 medium vine-ripened tomatoes, halved crosswise

1 tablespoon extra-virgin olive oil

1/4 teaspoon sea salt, divided

5 cups packed fresh leafy greens of choice, such as tatsoi (5 ounces)

5 cups packed fresh baby spinach (5 ounces)

Juice of 1/2 small lemon (1 tablespoon)

1/8 teaspoon freshly grated or ground nutmeg

3/4 cup Hollandaise-Style Sauce, warm (page 21)

1/8 teaspoon ground sumac or cayenne pepper, or to taste

1. Preheat the oven to 450°F. Brush the cauliflower slices and tomato halves with the oil, and arrange on a large baking sheet lined with unbleached parchment paper. Roast until the cauliflower and tomato halves are lightly caramelized, about 20 minutes. Gently flip over just the cauliflower. Sprinkle the cauliflower and tomato halves with 1/8 teaspoon salt. Roast until the cauliflower is fully caramelized and tomatoes are fully roasted, about 18 minutes more.

2. Meanwhile, add the leafy greens and spinach to a stockpot or large, deep skillet over medium heat. Cover and steam until all greens are fully wilted, about 8 minutes, stirring twice. (Note: The greens will wilt down to about 1 1/3 cups.) Add the lemon juice, nutmeg, and the remaining 1/8 teaspoon salt. Transfer the greens to a fine-mesh strainer to gently drain excess liquids.

3. Top each cauliflower slice with about 1/3 cup greens, a roasted tomato half, and 3 tablespoons sauce. Sprinkle with the sumac. Serve immediately.

*With a chef's knife, slice down from the top of the cauliflower head through the stem end. If you're unable to find a large head of cauliflower (2 pounds or larger), use 2 medium heads and cut slices slightly thicker. Use the largest center slices for this dish.

{ WITH POULTRY, FISH, OR MEAT }

One serving: In step 3, top one of the cauliflower slices with a 1/2-ounce thin slice of pan-grilled smoked chicken breast or turkey pastrami before topping with the greens.

Full recipe: Top each cauliflower slice with a 1/2-ounce thin slice of smoked chicken breast or turkey pastrami about 8 minutes before the end of the roasting process in step 1.

without
Exchanges/Food Choices: 1 Carbohydrate, 2 Vegetable, 1 Fat
160 calories, 70 calories from fat, 7g total fat, 1g saturated fat, 0g trans fat, 0mg cholesterol, 490mg sodium, 460mg potassium, 20g total carbohydrate, 9g dietary fiber, 6g sugars, 8g protein, 90mg phosphorus

with
Exchanges/Food Choices: 1 Carbohydrate, 2 Vegetable, 1 1/2 Fat
170 calories, 70 calories from fat, 8g total fat, 1g saturated fat, 0g trans fat, 10mg cholesterol, 580mg sodium, 490mg potassium, 20g total carbohydrate, 9g dietary fiber, 6g sugars, 10g protein, 120mg phosphorus

Hollandaise-Style Sauce

Makes 4 servings: 3 tablespoons each

1/2 cup silken tofu, drained

2 tablespoons plain unsweetened almond milk or other plant-based milk

Juice and zest of 1 small lemon (2 tablespoons juice)

1 tablespoon raw no-salt-added creamy almond butter

1 1/2 teaspoons spicy Dijon or brown mustard

3/4 teaspoon vegetarian Worcestershire sauce, or to taste

1/4 teaspoon hot Madras curry powder, or to taste

1/4 teaspoon sea salt, or to taste

1. Add the tofu, almond milk, lemon juice, almond butter, mustard, Worcestershire sauce, curry powder, and salt to a blender. Cover and purée until smooth.

2. Pour the tofu mixture into a small saucepan over medium heat. Simmer while stirring until fully heated, about 3 minutes. Stir in desired amount of the lemon zest and adjust seasoning. If preferred, reserve some of the zest for garnishing. Serve while warm in Roasted Cauliflower Florentine. Makes 3/4 cup.

Exchanges/Food Choices: 1/2 Fat
45 calories, 25 calories from fat, 3g total fat, 0g saturated fat, 0g trans fat, 0mg cholesterol, 210mg sodium, 50mg potassium, 3g total carbohydrate, 1g dietary fiber, 1g sugars, 2g protein, 20mg phosphorus

Sunrise Scrambled Squash and Poblano Tacos

Makes 4 servings: 2 tacos each

3/4 cup guacamole of choice
   (page 159)

8 (6-inch) soft whole-grain corn
   tortillas

1 tablespoon canola or unrefined
   peanut oil

3 scallions, green and white parts,
   thinly sliced

2 medium (7 ounces each) zucchini or
   yellow squash, finely diced

1 large (4.5-ounce) Poblano pepper,
   minced

1 (14-ounce) package extra-firm
   or firm tofu, drained and gently
   squeezed of excess liquid, finely
   diced*

1 teaspoon ground cumin

1/2 teaspoon finely chopped fresh
   oregano leaves

1/2 teaspoon sea salt, or to taste

1/4 teaspoon ground turmeric

1 cup cherry tomatoes, quartered

Juice of 1/2 lime (1 tablespoon)

3 tablespoons chopped fresh cilantro
   and 8 fresh cilantro sprigs

This recipe provides a sneaky way to add tofu. Here it's kind of like scrambled eggs, but it makes a perfect filling for tortillas. All of the herbs and spices create so much aroma and flavor appeal, you might turn tofu likers into lovers. What's more, these stuffed soft tacos (you get two for a serving!) create a fully satisfying meal on their own. Use a combination of zucchini and yellow squash for added interest. The triple combination of protein, fiber, and veggie volume will carry you through to lunch. In fact, enjoy these for lunch, too!

1. Spread 1 1/2 tablespoons guacamole onto each tortilla. Set aside.

2. Heat the oil in a large skillet over medium-high heat. Add the scallions, zucchini, and Poblano pepper, and sauté for 2 minutes.

3. Add the tofu, cumin, oregano, salt, and turmeric, and sauté until the zucchini is tender, about 8 minutes. Stir in the tomatoes and lime juice, and sauté until the tomatoes are heated through, about 2 minutes. Stir in the chopped cilantro. Adjust seasoning.

4. Spoon about 1/2 cup tofu mixture down the center of each tortilla. Top each tortilla with a cilantro sprig, fold, and serve.

*Or for an extra flavor kick, try with extra-firm spinach-jalapeño-flavored tofu.

One serving: Heat 1/2 teaspoon canola or unrefined peanut oil in a small, nonstick skillet over medium-high heat. Add 1 ounce ground turkey (about 94% lean) and sauté until well crumbled and fully cooked, about 2 minutes. Stir in 1 1/2 tablespoons tomatillo salsa (salsa verde) or other salsa, and cook while stirring until no excess liquid remains, about 2 minutes. Arrange the turkey down the center of 2 tortillas after spreading with the guacamole in step 1.

Full recipe: Heat 2 teaspoons canola or unrefined peanut oil in a large, nonstick skillet over medium-high heat. Add 4 ounces ground turkey (about 94% lean) and sauté until well crumbled and fully cooked, about 2 minutes. Stir in 1/4 cup plus 2 tablespoons tomatillo salsa (salsa verde) or other salsa, and cook while stirring until no excess liquid remains, about 2 minutes. Arrange the turkey down the center of each tortilla after spreading with the guacamole in step 1.

without
Exchanges/Food Choices: 1 1/2 Starch, 2 Vegetable, 1 Lean Meat, 2 Fat
310 calories, 140 calories from fat, 16g total fat, 2g saturated fat, 0g trans fat, 0mg cholesterol, 410mg sodium, 530mg potassium, 31g total carbohydrate, 9g dietary fiber, 5g sugars, 15g protein, 180mg phosphorus

with
Exchanges/Food Choices: 1 1/2 Starch, 2 Vegetable, 2 Lean Meat, 3 Fat
380 calories, 180 calories from fat, 21g total fat, 3g saturated fat, 0g trans fat, 20mg cholesterol, 590mg sodium, 530mg potassium, 32g total carbohydrate, 9g dietary fiber, 5g sugars, 21g protein, 230mg phosphorus

Corn, Canola, and Soy: Should You Go Organic?

Most of the corn, canola, and soybeans produced in the U.S. is genetically modified—otherwise known as GMO. The details are murky regarding the negative health effects and long-term safety of GMO-produced foods. There is so much we still don't know. I'm concerned enough about this production method that I prefer to be cautious. When purchasing corn, canola, and soy foods, I generally choose certified organic picks—which means they'll be free of GMOs. Something else you can look for is a Non-GMO Project Verified seal. It may not always be possible to choose these non-GMO or organic corn, canola, or soy foods due to availability or cost. But it's something to consider as an added step in your quest for optimal health.

Fruit Crepes with Summery Herb Salad

Makes 4 servings: 2 crepes each

3/4 cup plain almond unsweetened milk or other plant-based milk

1 large organic egg

1 tablespoon canola or extra-virgin olive oil, divided

1 teaspoon chopped fresh rosemary, or to taste

1/4 teaspoon + 1/8 teaspoon sea salt

1/2 cup buckwheat flour

3/4 cup shredded vegan mozzarella cheese alternative or part-skim mozzarella cheese

1/3 cup finely crumbed goat cheese or gorgonzola cheese (1.5 ounces)

3/4 cup thinly sliced fresh strawberries or fresh Black Mission figs

3/4 teaspoon freshly ground black pepper, or to taste

3 cups packed fresh herb salad or baby greens (3 ounces)

1/8 cup extra-thinly sliced red onion

2 teaspoons aged or white balsamic vinegar

Crepes may look like thin pancakes, but they're so much more interesting since you can fill them with nearly any savory or sweet ingredient. Or you can have the best of both food worlds, like I did here. By using a mixture of a vegan cheese and creamy goat cheese, you'll get cheesy goodness in a heart-friendlier way. Then, the sweet part comes into play. In early summer, choose strawberries with goat cheese; in late summer, go for figs with gorgonzola. All wrapped up, and served with crisp salad greens, this is a lovely item for brunch.

1. Whisk together the almond milk, egg, 2 teaspoons oil, the rosemary, and 1/4 teaspoon salt in a medium bowl. Add the flour and whisk vigorously until the mixture is very smooth, about 1 minute. Let the batter stand for 15 minutes.

2. Heat a nonstick crepe pan over medium heat. Spoon about 2 rounded tablespoons batter into the pan, tilting the pan to make a thin circular crepe. Cook until the crepe is done on the bottom, about 1 1/2 minutes.

3. Flip over, top with 1 rounded tablespoon mozzarella cheese, 1 rounded teaspoon goat cheese, 1 rounded tablespoon strawberries, and pinch of the pepper, and cook until done, about 1 1/2 minutes. Roll into a cone shape and arrange on a heatproof platter. Repeat the process with the remaining batter, cheeses, strawberries, and pepper to make 8 crepes. Keep warm in a 200°F oven, if necessary.

4. Toss together the salad greens, onion, vinegar, and the remaining 1 teaspoon oil and 1/8 teaspoon salt in a medium bowl. Arrange the salad on top or alongside of the crepes, and serve.

{ WITH POULTRY, FISH, OR MEAT }

One serving: Top 2 crepes with 1/2 ounce each thinly sliced smoked turkey breast before the strawberries in step 3.

Full recipe: Top all 8 crepes with 1/2 ounce each thinly sliced smoked turkey breast before the strawberries in step 3.

without
Exchanges/Food Choices: 1/2 Starch, 2 Fat
190 calories, 100 calories from fat, 12g total fat, 2.5g saturated fat, 0g trans fat, 50mg cholesterol, 360mg sodium, 260mg potassium, 14g total carbohydrate, 4g dietary fiber, 4g sugars, 7g protein, 70mg phosphorus

with
Exchanges/Food Choices: 1/2 Starch, 1 Medium-Fat Meat, 2 Fat
210 calories, 110 calories from fat, 12g total fat, 2.5g saturated fat, 0g trans fat, 65mg cholesterol, 580mg sodium, 320mg potassium, 15g total carbohydrate, 4g dietary fiber, 5g sugars, 13g protein, 120mg phosphorus

Portabella, Rosemary Egg White, and Greens Panini

1/2 Hass avocado, peeled, pitted, and cubed

1 1/2 teaspoons fresh lemon juice, divided

2 whole-grain sandwich rounds (thins), split

2 teaspoons canola or extra-virgin olive oil, divided

6 large organic egg whites or 3/4 cup pasteurized 100% egg whites

1 teaspoon finely chopped fresh rosemary or tarragon

1/8 teaspoon sea salt, or to taste

2 large (5-inch) portabella mushroom caps

1/2 teaspoon freshly ground black pepper

3/4 cup packed fresh mizuna, baby arugula, or mesclun (0.75 ounce)

Get your grill on in the morning! Making a bountiful egg-white panini sandwich filled with the best ingredients will help start your day off in style. The best part is the portabella because it provides body and meatiness. When available, choose UV-grown portabellas (that means they're exposed to ultraviolet light) for a boost of vitamin D. Make this panini your number one breakfast pick for Saturdays. If you make it often, mix things up by trying it with various fresh herbs!

1. Mash the avocado with 1/2 teaspoon lemon juice in a small bowl. Arrange the sandwich rounds cut side up. Spread all of the rounds with the mashed avocado. Set aside.

2. Heat 1 teaspoon oil in a small nonstick skillet over medium heat. Add the egg whites and rosemary, and cook undisturbed until the bottom of the egg whites are firm and lightly browned on the bottom and no longer runny on the top, about 7 minutes. Flip the entire egg-white "omelet" over and cook until done, about 30 seconds. Transfer to a cutting board. Cut into 6 wedges, sprinkle with the salt, and set aside.

3. Preheat a panini grill on medium-high heat. Rub the rounded side of the mushroom caps with the remaining 1 teaspoon oil, then sprinkle the gill side with the pepper. Cook the mushroom caps in the panini grill with the gill side up, until fully cooked, about 4 minutes. Remove from the panini grill. Arrange 3 egg-white wedges onto each bottom sandwich round. Top with the grilled mushroom caps. Add the top sandwich rounds.

4. Cook the egg-white sandwiches in the panini grill until the sandwich rounds are lightly grilled, about 4 minutes.

5. Meanwhile, toss together the mizuna and the remaining 1 teaspoon lemon juice in a bowl. Insert the mizuna into the paninis, and serve.

{ WITH POULTRY, FISH, OR MEAT }

One serving: Cut the salt in the recipe by half (use just a pinch) and do not add salt to 3 egg white wedges in step 2. Place 1/3 ounce extra-thinly sliced prosciutto or American country ham on top of the grilled mushroom cap that's placed on the no-salt-added egg-white wedges, then add the sandwich top in step 3.

Full recipe: Remove the salt from the recipe. Place 1/3 ounce extra-thinly sliced prosciutto or American country ham on top of each grilled mushroom cap, then add sandwich tops.

Pinch and Smidgen

In a handful of recipes you'll see that I call for a pinch or smidgen of salt, pepper, or spice. If you like specifics, here's what I used as their equivalent:
Pinch = 1/16 teaspoon
Smidgen = 1/32 teaspoon

without
Exchanges/Food Choices: 1 Starch, 1 Vegetable, 1 Lean Meat, 2 Fat
260 calories, 100 calories from fat, 11g total fat, 1.5g saturated fat, 0g trans fat, 0mg cholesterol, 480mg sodium, 760mg potassium, 26g total carbohydrate, 7g dietary fiber, 6g sugars, 17g protein, 250mg phosphorus

with
Exchanges/Food Choices: 1 Starch, 1 Vegetable, 1 1/2 Lean Meat, 2 Fat
280 calories, 110 calories from fat, 12g total fat, 1.5g saturated fat, 0g trans fat, 5mg cholesterol, 590mg sodium, 810mg potassium, 26g total carbohydrate, 7g dietary fiber, 6g sugars, 20g protein, 280mg phosphorus

Heirloom Tomato, Arugula, and Over-Easy Egg Muffin

Makes 4 servings: 1 muffin sandwich each

4 (1/2-inch) thick slices large heirloom or vine-ripened tomato, patted dry (10 ounces total)

1/4 teaspoon sea salt, divided

8 large or 16 small fresh sage leaves

1 1/2 cups packed fresh baby or wild arugula (1.5 ounces)

2 teaspoons fresh lemon juice

4 whole-grain English muffins, split

1 1/2 teaspoons canola or extra-virgin olive oil

4 medium organic eggs

1/4 teaspoon freshly ground black pepper, or to taste

Move over, wimpy, greasy, drive-thru breakfast sandwich! This gorgeous sandwich will open up your eyes and taste buds to a brand new morning meal experience. A sage-roasted tomato and crisp, fresh arugula provide so much enticement when paired with a yolky egg. A word of caution: this stuffed sandwich is so super juicy that it may best be eaten with a fork and knife.

1. Preheat the oven to 450°F. Place tomato slices onto a baking pan lined with unbleached parchment paper. Sprinkle with 1/8 teaspoon salt and top with the sage leaves. Roast in the oven until cooked through, about 15 minutes. Remove from the oven.

2. Toss the arugula with the lemon juice in a small bowl; set aside. Lightly toast the English muffin halves. Place each sage-roasted tomato on the bottom muffin halves. Set aside.

3. Heat the oil in a large, nonstick skillet over medium heat. Break the eggs into the skillet, add the pepper and the remaining 1/8 teaspoon salt, and cook until the undersides of the eggs are firm, about 3 minutes. Gently flip each egg over and cook until the whites are firm and the yolks are still soft, about 1 minute.

4. Top each tomato slice with an egg. Top with the dressed arugula. Place the remaining muffin halves on top and serve.

{ WITH POULTRY, FISH, OR MEAT }

One serving: Add half of a 1/2-ounce slice of hot or sweet sopressata to one of the toasted muffin halves before topping with the tomato slice in step 2.

Full recipe: Add half of a 1/2-ounce slice of hot or sweet sopressata to each of the 4 toasted muffin halves before topping with the tomato slices in step 2.

without
Exchanges/Food Choices: 1 1/2 Starch, 1 Vegetable, 1 Fat
230 calories, 70 calories from fat, 8g total fat, 2g saturated fat, 0g trans fat, 165mg cholesterol, 460mg sodium, 410mg potassium, 31g total carbohydrate, 6g dietary fiber, 8g sugars, 12g protein, 300mg phosphorus

with
Exchanges/Food Choices: 1 1/2 Starch, 1 Vegetable, 1 Medium-Fat Meat, 1 Fat
260 calories, 90 calories from fat, 10g total fat, 2.5g saturated fat, 0g trans fat, 170mg cholesterol, 590mg sodium, 440mg potassium, 31g total carbohydrate, 6g dietary fiber, 8g sugars, 14g protein, 310mg phosphorus

Open-Face Bagel Thins with Scallion Schmear

Makes 2 servings: 2 open-face bagel thins each

1/4 cup plain fat-free Greek yogurt

2 tablespoons Neufchatel (light cream cheese), at room temperature

2 scallions, green and white parts, minced

2 teaspoons finely chopped fresh dill or tarragon, divided

1 teaspoon tiny capers, well drained

1 teaspoon fresh lime or lemon juice

1/4 teaspoon freshly ground black pepper, or to taste

1/8 teaspoon sea salt, or to taste

2 whole-grain "everything" or whole-wheat bagel thins, split and toasted*

Bagels are back...and thinner. It's only the big ol' bakery ones that can cause carb overload.Whole-grain bagel thins are the carb-friendlier answer to getting your bagel fix. Of course, you'll probably want to serve each toasty thin with a cream-cheesy spread, so I've created a naturally light topping by combining Neufchatel and Greek yogurt. Luckily the topping is anything but light on flavor due to the fresh scallions, fragrant herbs, and zingy capers.

1. Stir together the yogurt, Neufchatel, scallions, 1 teaspoon of the dill, the capers, lime juice, pepper, and salt in a small bowl until well combined. (Makes 1/2 cup.)

2. Dollop or spread the schmear, about 2 tablespoons each, onto the toasted bagel thins. Sprinkle with the remaining 1 teaspoon dill and serve.

*Alternatively, use 2 whole-grain "everything" bagels. Split them and pinch out the bready filling to form 4 bagel shells.

{ WITH POULTRY, FISH, OR MEAT }

One serving: Before adding the salt in step 1, transfer 1/4 cup schmear into a separate small bowl. Add only a pinch of salt to one of the bowls of schmear; do not add salt to the other bowl. After spreading the bagel thins with the schmears, top each of the bagel thin pieces containing the no-salt-added schmear with 1/2 ounce thinly sliced Scottish smoked salmon or turkey pastrami before sprinkling with the remaining dill in step 2.

Full recipe: Do not add salt to the schmear in step 1. After spreading each piece of bagel thin with the schmear, top each with 1/2 ounce thinly sliced Scottish smoked salmon or turkey pastrami, then sprinkle with the remaining dill in step 2.

without
Exchanges/Food Choices: 2 1/2 Starch, 1/2 Vegetable, 1/2 Fat
250 calories, 50 calories from fat, 6g total fat, 2g saturated fat, 0g trans fat, 10mg cholesterol, 470mg sodium, 280mg potassium, 45g total carbohydrate, 7g dietary fiber, 7g sugars, 11g protein, 300mg phosphorus

with
Exchanges/Food Choices: 2 1/2 Starch, 1/2 Vegetable, 1 Lean Meat, 1/2 Fat
280 calories, 60 calories from fat, 7g total fat, 2g saturated fat, 0g trans fat, 15mg cholesterol, 550mg sodium, 330mg potassium, 45g total carbohydrate, 7g dietary fiber, 6g sugars, 16g protein, 340mg phosphorus

British-Style Beans on Toast

Makes 1 serving: 1 topped toast

1/2 cup canned vegetarian baked beans in tomato sauce

1 slice low-sodium sprouted whole-grain bread or other whole-grain bread

2 teaspoons minced fresh chives

1/8 teaspoon freshly ground black pepper, or to taste

without
Exchanges/Food Choices: 2 1/2 Starch
200 calories, 10 calories from fat,
1g total fat, 0g saturated fat, 0g trans fat,
0mg cholesterol, 480mg sodium,
290mg potassium, 39g total carbohydrate,
9g dietary fiber, 9g sugars, 9g protein,
100mg phosphorus

with
Exchanges/Food Choices: 2 Starch,
1/2 Medium-Fat Meat
200 calories, 20 calories from fat,
2.5g total fat, 0g saturated fat, 0g trans fat,
25mg cholesterol, 520mg sodium,
230mg potassium, 31g total carbohydrate,
7g dietary fiber, 6g sugars, 13g protein,
110mg phosphorus

For a simple yet bold breakfast entrée, look no further. This high-flavor recipe is so satisfying, and it has a touch of sweetness to put a big smile on the face of bean lovers. The luscious beans add more interest to toast than butter ever could. It's extra tasty when the bread sops up the sauciness of the beans, but you can strain the beans if you prefer. Try this four-ingredient fix for dinner, too. It's both quick and delicious!

1. Simmer the beans according to can directions.

2. Toast or grill the bread.

3. Top the toast with the beans, chives, and pepper, and serve. Enjoy with a fork and knife.

{ WITH POULTRY, FISH, OR MEAT }

For one serving (full recipe): Top the toast with 1/3 cup beans instead of 1/2 cup. Then, top with one well-crisped, pan-cooked slice of hardwood-smoked, uncured turkey bacon or Sunday bacon. Sprinkle with the chives and pepper, and serve.

"Hash Browns"

Makes 4 servings: 1 cup each

There are no potatoes in this unique and tasty take on hash browns. It provides just 100 calories in an entire cupful. But it's not the calories that you'll be raving about. The skillet-browned cauliflower is the delectable star here. And the Serrano pepper gives it a memorable kick.

1. Heat the oil in a large, nonstick skillet over medium-high heat. Add the cauliflower, onion, Serrano pepper, vinegar, and 1/4 teaspoon salt. Stir to combine. Cover and cook until the cauliflower begins to caramelize, about 7 minutes, stirring twice during cooking.

2. Remove the lid and continue to sauté until the cauliflower is fully cooked and caramelized as desired. Add the scallions, garlic, rosemary, and the remaining 1/4 teaspoon salt, and sauté for 1 minute. Adjust seasoning.

3. Stir in or sprinkle with the parsley, and serve immediately.

WITH POULTRY, FISH, OR MEAT

One serving: Stir 1/4 ounce finely diced or minced Toscano-style dry salami or turkey salami into 1 cup "hash browns" when serving in step 3.

Full recipe: Stir 1 ounce finely diced or minced Toscano-style dry salami or turkey salami into the "hash browns" with the parsley in step 3.

1 1/2 tablespoons canola or extra-virgin olive oil

1 1/2 pounds small cauliflower florets (6 cups)

1 medium white onion, diced

1 Serrano pepper, with some seeds, minced

2 teaspoons white wine vinegar

1/2 teaspoon sea salt, divided

2 scallions, green and white parts, minced

2 large garlic cloves, minced

2 teaspoons finely chopped fresh rosemary or sage

1/4 cup roughly chopped fresh flat-leaf parsley

without
Exchanges/Food Choices: 2 Vegetable, 1 Fat
100 calories, 50 calories from fat, 6g total fat, 0.5g saturated fat, 0g trans fat, 0mg cholesterol, 320mg sodium, 330mg potassium, 11g total carbohydrate, 5g dietary fiber, 5g sugars, 4g protein, 70mg phosphorus

with
Exchanges/Food Choices: 2 Vegetable, 1 1/2 Fat
130 calories, 80 calories from fat, 9g total fat, 1.5g saturated fat, 0g trans fat, 5mg cholesterol, 480mg sodium, 360mg potassium, 11g total carbohydrate, 5g dietary fiber, 5g sugars, 5g protein, 90mg phosphorus

Winter Vegetable Hash

Makes 4 servings: about 1 cup each

1 tablespoon canola or extra-virgin
    olive oil

1 large (9-ounce) red onion, diced

1 medium (7-ounce) sweet potato,
    unpeeled, cut into 1/4-inch cubes

1 1/2 cups chopped broccoli florets
    and tender stems

1 tablespoon white wine vinegar,
    divided

1/2 teaspoon freshly ground black
    pepper, or to taste

1/4 teaspoon + 1/8 teaspoon sea salt,
    or to taste

3 vegetarian breakfast "sausage"
    patties

1 teaspoon finely chopped fresh
    rosemary

3 cups packed fresh baby spinach
    (3 ounces)

Traditional hash is made with chopped meat, potatoes or other vegetables, and spices. But for an unconventional taste tempter, stir up this flavorful recipe. It's light on calories, yet it's a truly filling entrée thanks to all the veggies. For an extra palate-friendly, eye-popping option, top each serving with a medium-size organic poached egg. This recipe proves that not sticking with tradition can be a very good thing.

1. Heat the oil in a large, nonstick skillet over medium heat. Add the onion, sweet potato, broccoli, 1 teaspoon vinegar, the pepper, and 1/4 teaspoon salt; cover, and cook until the sweet potato and broccoli are tender and onion is lightly caramelized, about 15 minutes, stirring once.

2. Meanwhile, prepare the breakfast "sausage" patties according to package directions. Finely dice. Set aside and keep warm.

3. Uncover the skillet, add the rosemary, and sauté until the onion and sweet potato are fully caramelized, about 5 minutes. Add the spinach and the remaining 2 teaspoons vinegar and 1/8 teaspoon salt, and stir until fully wilted, about 1 1/2 minutes. Stir in the "sausage" and adjust seasoning.

4. Divide the hash among individual plates, and serve.

{ WITH POULTRY, FISH, OR MEAT }

One serving: Separately, prepare a 1 1/2-ounce portion of a fully cooked sweet Italian poultry link according to package directions instead of one of the vegetarian patties in step 2. Thinly slice or finely dice the sausage and keep warm in a small skillet. Before stirring in the "sausage" in step 3, transfer 3/4 cup (one serving without "sausage") of the hash to the small skillet and stir into the sausage.

Full recipe: Prepare 6 ounces fully cooked sweet Italian poultry links according to package directions instead of the 3 breakfast "sausage" patties in step 2.

without
Exchanges/Food Choices: 1 Starch, 1 Vegetable, 1/2 Fat
170 calories, 60 calories from fat, 7g total fat, 0g saturated fat, 0g trans fat, 0mg cholesterol, 560mg sodium, 330mg potassium, 19g total carbohydrate, 5g dietary fiber, 5g sugars, 10g protein, 50mg phosphorus

with
Exchanges/Food Choices: 1 Starch, 1 Vegetable, 1 Medium-Fat Meat, 1/2 Fat
170 calories, 60 calories from fat, 7g total fat, 1.3g saturated fat, 0g trans fat, 35mg cholesterol, 520mg sodium, 410mg potassium, 17g total carbohydrate, 4g dietary fiber, 5g sugars, 10g protein, 130mg phosphorus

Gouda Grits with Greens

Makes 8 servings: 1/2 cup grits with 1/4 cup greens each

1 1/4 cups plain unsweetened almond milk or other plant-based milk

3/4 teaspoon sea salt, or to taste

1 cup yellow corn grits (polenta; not instant)

1/4 cup plain fat-free Greek yogurt, at room temperature

1 teaspoon unsalted butter, at room temperature

1/4 cup shredded extra-aged Boerenkaas or aged Gouda cheese (1 ounce)

2 cups packed tatsoi, mâche, or watercress leaves (2 ounces)

1/2 small lemon, cut into 8 wedges (optional)

Sometimes you need to sacrifice style when going for comfort. That's not the case with this chic and cozy side dish. The grits get their creaminess from plant-based milk, Greek yogurt, and even a touch of real butter. Then, each dish is accented with shreds of a tangy cheese and accessorized with intriguing fresh greens. It's a side that will be the center of attention.

1. Bring 2 cups water, the almond milk, and salt to a boil in a large saucepan over high heat. Slowly stir in the grits until thoroughly combined, and return to a boil. Reduce heat to low and cook while stirring until thickened, about 3 minutes. (Note: The mixture will splatter slightly.) Remove from heat. Stir in the yogurt and butter until well combined and the butter is fully melted. Adjust seasoning.

2. Immediately transfer the grits to individual bowls and sprinkle with the Boerenkaas cheese and tatsoi. Serve with the optional lemon wedges and enjoy immediately.

{ WITH POULTRY, FISH, OR MEAT }

One serving: Insert 4 medium peeled and deveined shrimp onto a metal or water-soaked bamboo skewer. Brush with about 1/2 teaspoon grapeseed or canola oil. Grill or pan-grill over direct medium-high heat until just cooked through, about 1 1/2–2 minutes per side. Sprinkle with a pinch of Cajun or Creole seasoning. Place onto one of the servings of grits after the tatsoi in step 2.

Full recipe: Insert 32 medium peeled and deveined shrimp onto 8 metal or water-soaked bamboo skewers, 4 per skewer. Brush with 1 tablespoon grapeseed or canola oil. Grill or pan-grill over direct medium-high heat until just cooked through, about 1 1/2–2 minutes per side. Sprinkle with 1/2 teaspoon of Cajun or Creole seasoning. Place a shrimp skewer onto each serving of grits after the tatsoi in step 2.

without
Exchanges/Food Choices: 1 Starch, 1/2 Fat
100 calories, 20 calories from fat, 2g total fat,
1g saturated fat, 0g trans fat, 5mg cholesterol,
280mg sodium, 100mg potassium, 18g total
carbohydrate, 1g dietary fiber, 1g sugars,
3g protein, 40mg phosphorus

with
Exchanges/Food Choices: 1 Starch, 1 Lean Meat,
1/2 Fat
130 calories, 35 calories from fat, 4g total fat,
1g saturated fat, 0g trans fat, 30mg cholesterol,
430mg sodium, 120mg potassium, 18g total
carbohydrate, 1g dietary fiber, 1g sugars,
6g protein, 90mg phosphorus

CHAPTER 2

starters and snacks

Peanut Salad in Wonton Cups

Makes 8 servings: 3 stuffed wonton cups each

24 square whole-grain wonton wrappers

1 tablespoon canola or unrefined peanut oil, divided

1 tablespoon creamy no-salt-added natural peanut butter

1 tablespoon no-sugar-added apple or apple-peach sauce

2 teaspoons fresh lime juice

1 1/2 teaspoons naturally brewed soy sauce

1 teaspoon spicy Dijon mustard

1 teaspoon freshly grated gingerroot

2 1/2 cups packed finely shredded Romaine hearts

1 small or 1/2 large red bell pepper, finely diced

2 scallions, green and white parts, thinly sliced on the diagonal

1 tablespoon chopped fresh cilantro

2 tablespoons chopped unsalted roasted peanuts

No utensils are required for this Asian-inspired hors d'oeuvre salad. But do serve with a plate, as the salad is nearly overstuffed into petite wonton cups. The Romaine creates freshness, and the dressing adds perkiness. These crisp salad cups will be a hit at any get-together.

1. Preheat the oven to 325°F. Very lightly rub or brush both sides of the wonton wrappers with 2 teaspoons oil. Press a wonton wrapper into each cup of a mini-muffin tin with 24 cups (or 2 tins with 12 cups each). Bake until deep golden brown and crisp, about 15 minutes, rotating tray(s) halfway through baking and gently reforming any cups that might have slightly collapsed inward during the beginning part of the baking process. Cool on a rack.

2. Whisk together the peanut butter, applesauce, lime juice, soy sauce, mustard, ginger, and the remaining 1 teaspoon oil in a medium bowl.

3. Just before serving, toss together the Romaine hearts, bell pepper, scallions, and cilantro in a large bowl. Add the peanut butter dressing and toss to coat. Adjust seasoning. (Makes about 3 cups.)

4. Stuff each wonton cup with about 2 tablespoons salad, sprinkle with the peanuts, and serve immediately. (Note: The salad will get soggy if you make these in advance.)

{ WITH POULTRY, FISH, OR MEAT }

One serving: Toss 2 tablespoons finely diced grilled or roasted chicken thigh meat with 1/8 teaspoon naturally brewed soy sauce in a small bowl. In step 3, transfer 1/3 cup dressed salad to the small bowl with the chicken, and toss. Pack into 3 wonton cups and continue with step 4.

Full recipe: In step 2, stir 1 cup finely diced grilled or roasted chicken thigh meat and an additional 1 teaspoon naturally brewed soy sauce into the peanut butter dressing in the medium bowl.

without
Exchanges/Food Choices: 1 Starch,
1 Vegetable, 1 Fat
120 calories, 40 calories from fat, 4.5g total
fat, 0.5g saturated fat, 0g trans fat, 0mg
cholesterol, 210mg sodium, 130mg potassium,
17g total carbohydrate, 1g dietary fiber,
1g sugars, 4g protein, 50mg phosphorus

with
Exchanges/Food Choices: 1 Starch,
1 Vegetable, 1 Lean Meat, 1 Fat
150 calories, 50 calories from fat, 6g total fat,
1g saturated fat, 0g trans fat, 25mg cholesterol,
270mg sodium, 170mg potassium, 17g total
carbohydrate, 1g dietary fiber, 1g sugars,
8g protein, 80mg phosphorus

Pan-Grilled Tofu Skewers

Makes 6 servings: 3 skewers each

2 tablespoons naturally brewed soy sauce

1 1/2 tablespoons brown rice vinegar

1 scallion, green and white parts, minced

1 tablespoon freshly grated gingerroot

1 tablespoon no-sugar-added apple-apricot sauce or applesauce

2 teaspoons toasted sesame oil

1/4 teaspoon dried hot pepper flakes

1 (14-ounce) package extra-firm tofu, drained and squeezed of excess liquid

1 teaspoon black or white sesame seeds (or a mixture), toasted

2 tablespoons fresh small cilantro leaves

If you're looking for an introduction to tofu, meet these Szechuan skewers. They offer a tasty way to try tofu for the first time, or the 101st time! Marinated in a gingery vinaigrette, inserted onto skewers, grilled until lovely caramelized grill markings form, and garnished with fresh cilantro leaves and sesame seeds, these tofu "pops" will be a hit for all the senses. Try them at your next cook-in... or cookout!

1. Whisk together the soy sauce, vinegar, scallion, ginger, apple-apricot sauce, sesame oil, and hot pepper flakes in a small bowl. (Makes 1/2 cup.) Pour into a 9 × 13-inch pan or similar-size dish.

2. Cut the tofu lengthwise into 9 slices; then, cut each slice in half lengthwise or crosswise, creating 18 pieces. Place the tofu slices in a single layer in the soy sauce mixture and marinate about 10–15 minutes per side.

3. Preheat a grill pan over medium-high heat. Transfer each tofu slice to the pan using tongs, reserving the marinade. Grill (in batches) until deep grill marks form on both sides, about 3 1/2–4 minutes per side.

4. Insert reusable or bamboo skewers into the cooked tofu, sprinkle with the sesame seeds and cilantro leaves, and serve while warm with the remaining marinade on the side.

{ WITH POULTRY, FISH, OR MEAT }

One serving: Use about 12 ounces (instead of 14 ounces) tofu cut into 15 pieces in step 2. Transfer 1 tablespoon + 1 teaspoon of the marinade to a small dish. Add 3 (3/4-ounce) pieces of boneless, skinless chicken thigh to the small dish and marinate for about 10–15 minutes per side. Grill until well done after the tofu in step 3. Do not reuse any remaining marinade from the uncooked chicken.

Full recipe: Instead of the tofu, use 18 (3/4-ounce) pieces of boneless, skinless chicken thigh and marinate for about 10–15 minutes per side. Grill until well done in step 3. Do not reuse any remaining marinade from the uncooked chicken.

without

Exchanges/Food Choices: 1 Medium-Fat Meat
90 calories, 50 calories from fat, 6g total fat, 0.5g saturated fat, 0g trans fat, 0mg cholesterol, 310mg sodium, 100mg potassium, 3g total carbohydrate, 1g dietary fiber, 1g sugars, 7g protein, 90mg phosphorus

with

Exchanges/Food Choices: 2 Lean Meat
100 calories, 50 calories from fat, 5g total fat, 1g saturated fat, 0g trans fat, 60mg cholesterol, 350mg sodium, 140mg potassium, 1g total carbohydrate, 0g dietary fiber, 1g sugars, 11g protein, 100mg phosphorus

Pesto-Glazed Vegetable Kebabs

Makes 6 servings: 2 skewers each

2 tablespoons basil pesto

2 tablespoons low-sodium vegetable broth or unsweetened green tea

1 large garlic clove, minced (optional)

1/4 teaspoon sea salt, divided

1 large yellow squash, scrubbed, and cut lengthwise in half; cut each half into 12 half moons

1 large zucchini, unpeeled, and cut lengthwise in half; cut each half into 12 half moons

8 ounces extra-firm pesto- or Italian-flavor tofu, cut into 24 cubes

1/4 teaspoon freshly ground black pepper, or to taste

6 fresh basil sprigs

Pesto is one of those decadent ingredients considered to be good for you, but in dainty dollops. I've "stretched" it here by using broth or unsweetened tea. It nicely coats the summery veggies in these kebabs. The culinary scene-stealer is the naturally flavored tofu interspersed among the zucchini and yellow squash. The tofu is already marinated, so all you need to do here is simply grill it. However, if you're unable to find flavored tofu, small white button mushroom caps are delicious, too.

1. Prepare an indoor or outdoor grill. Whisk together the pesto, broth, garlic (if using), and 1/8 teaspoon salt in a medium bowl. Add the yellow squash and zucchini and toss until coated.

2. Secure the vegetables and tofu cubes onto 12 (8-inch) reusable or water-soaked bamboo skewers, placing 2 pieces of yellow squash, 2 pieces of zucchini, and 2 cubes of tofu on each, preferably in alternating style.

3. Grill over direct medium-high heat until cooked through and grill marks form, about 3 1/2 minutes per side.

4. Sprinkle the kebabs with the pepper and the remaining 1/8 teaspoon salt. Adjust seasoning. Garnish each serving with a fresh basil sprig, and serve while warm or at room temperature.

{ WITH POULTRY, FISH, OR MEAT }

One serving: Cut about a 1-ounce piece of grass-fed, lean beef tenderloin or boneless sirloin into 4 cubes. Sprinkle with a smidgen of salt. Insert the 4 beef cubes onto 2 skewers instead of 1 ounce tofu in step 2.

Full recipe: Cut a 7-ounce grass-fed, lean beef tenderloin or boneless sirloin steak into 24 cubes. Sprinkle with 1/8 teaspoon sea salt. Insert 2 beef cubes onto each of the 12 skewers instead of the tofu in step 2.

without
Exchanges/Food Choices: 1 Vegetable, 1 Fat
100 calories, 50 calories from fat, 6g total fat, 1.5g saturated fat, 0g trans fat, 0mg cholesterol, 250mg sodium, 370mg potassium, 6g total carbohydrate, 2g dietary fiber, 3g sugars, 8g protein, 140mg phosphorus

with
Exchanges/Food Choices: 1 Vegetable, 1 Lean Meat, 1/2 Fat
90 calories, 40 calories from fat, 4.5g total fat, 1.5g saturated fat, 0g trans fat, 20mg cholesterol, 210mg sodium, 380mg potassium, 4g total carbohydrate, 1g dietary fiber, 2g sugars, 9g protein, 110mg phosphorus

Oven-Fried Nuggets

Makes 6 servings: 3 nuggets with marinara each

18 (2-inch diameter) crimini mushrooms

3/4 cup low-fat buttermilk

1 teaspoon freshly ground black pepper, divided

1/2 teaspoon + 1/8 teaspoon sea salt, or to taste

2 large garlic cloves, minced

3/4 teaspoon hot pepper sauce, or to taste

3/4 cup stone-ground whole-wheat flour

4 large organic egg whites or 1/2 cup pasteurized 100% egg whites

1 cup whole-wheat panko bread crumbs

Cooking spray

1 1/2 teaspoons herbes de Provence, or to taste

1/2 cup marinara sauce of choice, warm (page 191)

One of the ultimate family-friendly finger foods is chicken nuggets. Luckily, there's a veggie that makes a "meaty," and maybe more memorable, nugget: the crimini mushroom. You can have so much fun with this versatile recipe. Call these "'shroom poppers" if you like. Try other dipping sauces, such as tzatziki (page 175) instead of marinara, and serve these scrumptious bites as the starring ingredient in other recipes, like the Po' Boy-Inspired Sandwich (page 144).

1. Remove the mushroom stems; save the stems for another recipe, such as Gingery Asparagus, Couscous, and Crimini Soup (page 112). Preheat the oven to 450°F.

2. Add the buttermilk, 1/2 teaspoon black pepper, 1/4 teaspoon salt, the garlic, and hot sauce to a medium bowl. In a second bowl add the flour. In a third bowl whisk together the egg whites with 2 tablespoons cold water. In a fourth bowl add the panko. Dip each entire mushroom cap into the buttermilk mixture, then the flour, the egg-white mixture, and the panko, shaking off excess between each dip.

3. Place the coated crimini caps, rounded side up, onto a large baking sheet. Coat with cooking spray. Sprinkle with the herbes de Provence, 1/4 teaspoon salt, and the remaining 1/2 teaspoon black pepper. Bake until cooked through and the coating is brown and crisp, about 20 minutes, flipping over each cap about halfway through baking. Sprinkle with the remaining 1/8 teaspoon salt. Adjust seasoning.

4. Serve the nuggets while warm on a platter, rounded side up, with the marinara on the side.

{ WITH POULTRY, FISH, OR MEAT }

One serving: In place of 3 crimini caps, cut 1 1/2 ounces boneless, skinless, chicken breast into 3 cubes and dip into each of the mixtures after the mushroom caps in step 2. Bake on a separate small baking dish.

Full recipe: In place of all crimini caps, cut 9 ounces boneless, skinless, chicken breast into 18 cubes and dip into each of the mixtures in step 2. For best results, let the chicken marinate in the buttermilk mixture for about 30 minutes before dipping into the flour mixture.

without

Exchanges/Food Choices: 1 Starch, 1 Vegetable
110 calories, 10 calories from fat, 1g total fat,
0g saturated fat, 0g trans fat, 0mg cholesterol,
440mg sodium, 370mg potassium, 20g total
carbohydrate, 3g dietary fiber, 3g sugars,
6g protein, 90mg phosphorus

with

Exchanges/Food Choices: 1 Starch, 1 Lean Meat
140 calories, 15 calories from fat, 2g total fat,
0g saturated fat, 0g trans fat, 25mg cholesterol,
460mg sodium, 180mg potassium, 18g total
carbohydrate, 3g dietary fiber, 2g sugars,
13g protein, 90mg phosphorus

For Best Results When Breading

Try to keep one hand as the "dry" one and one as the "wet" hand during the entire breading process. In Oven-Fried Nuggets, you will not use up all of the buttermilk mixture, flour, or egg whites, but these amounts are recommended for best breading results.

Ancient Grain Grape Leaves

1 1/3 cups whole-grain (brown) teff or amaranth

3/4 cup minced sweet onion

1/4 cup finely chopped fresh flat-leaf parsley

1/4 cup finely chopped fresh mint

2 large garlic cloves, minced

1 1/4 teaspoons sea salt, or to taste

3/4 teaspoon freshly ground black pepper

1/2 teaspoon ground cinnamon

1/4 teaspoon ground allspice

30 large fresh grape leaves, lightly blanched, or grape leaves from jar, soaked in water, rinsed well, and drained

1 tablespoon extra-virgin olive oil

2 lemons

1 cup plain fat-free Greek yogurt

This stuffed grape leaves recipe is loosely based on the long-established Lebanese version that my mother taught me and her mother taught her. I added my own modern touch, however, using an ancient ingredient: teff. It's kind of like a culinary oxymoron with enticing results. Though botanically a cereal grass, teff is considered to be a nutrient-packed whole grain that's tiny, tasty, and gluten-free. It also has resistant starch, which is like a dietary fiber that may help with managing blood glucose and weight. Mostly, teff provides a curiously good filling for grape leaves.

1. Stir together the teff, onion, parsley, mint, garlic, salt, pepper, cinnamon, allspice, and 1/4 cup water in a medium mixing bowl. Set aside. (Makes 2 1/4 cups teff mixture.)

2. Lay the grape leaves individually, dull/vein side up, on unbleached paper towels. Snip off any long stems. Place about 1 rounded tablespoon teff mixture down the center of each leaf (like it's a burrito). Roll each leaf tightly by folding the bottom end of each leaf over the filling, folding the edges over the filling, then rolling toward the leaf point, until they look like mini green burritos.

3. After rolling each leaf, place seam side down, in a 10- or 11-inch heavy-duty skillet, firmly packing them in a single layer. Drizzle with the oil. Slowly pour water (about 2 1/4 cups) over the rolls until just covered.

4. Cut one of the lemons into small wedges and set aside. Squeeze the other lemon, creating about 3 tablespoons juice, and drizzle it over the stuffed grape leaves.

5. Place a heavy, heatproof plate onto the stuffed leaves to keep them from opening up during cooking. Place the skillet over high heat and bring to a boil. Cover, reduce heat to low, and cook until the teff is tender, about 1 hour, carefully removing the plate halfway through the cooking process. Remove from the heat, uncover, and let stand to complete the cooking process, about 15 minutes.

6. Arrange the stuffed grape leaves with the yogurt and reserved lemon wedges on a platter. Serve while warm or at room temperature.

{ WITH POULTRY, FISH, OR MEAT }

One serving: Not recommended

For full recipe: In step 1, prepare the mixture with 1 cup teff instead of 1 1/3 cups. Add 8 ounces raw, lean, ground, grass-fed beef sirloin or ground lamb to the teff mixture and combine by hand. Makes 2 1/2 cups teff-meat mixture.

without
Exchanges/Food Choices: 1 Starch, 1 Vegetable
140 calories, 30 calories from fat, 3.5g total fat, 0.5g saturated fat, 0g trans fat, 0mg cholesterol, 300mg sodium, 200mg potassium, 21g total carbohydrate, 3g dietary fiber, 3g sugars, 6g protein, 160mg phosphorus

with
Exchanges/Food Choices: 1 Starch, 1 Vegetable, 1 Lean Meat
140 calories, 35 calories from fat, 4g total fat, 1g saturated fat, 0g trans fat, 15mg cholesterol, 320mg sodium, 240mg potassium, 17g total carbohydrate, 3g dietary fiber, 3g sugars, 10g protein, 170mg phosphorus

Steamed Edamame Dumplings

Makes 8 servings: 3 dumplings each

1 1/2 cups frozen shelled edamame (7 ounces)

1 tablespoon hoisin sauce

2 teaspoons toasted sesame oil

1 1/2 teaspoons naturally brewed soy sauce

1/4 teaspoon dried hot pepper flakes

3 scallions, green and white parts, minced

2 teaspoons freshly grated gingerroot

1 large garlic clove, minced

1 tablespoon finely chopped fresh cilantro

24 round dumpling wrappers, preferably whole-wheat

Cooking spray

Edamame was relatively unknown by most until recently. Yet most still haven't used it in many culinary applications. So here you go. The edamame is pureed with exceptionally high-flavored Asian ingredients to create a memorable dumpling filling. Enjoy the dumplings simply as is or pair them with a dipping sauce, such as Gochujang, soy sauce, or a mixture of the two. They're equally delicious in Szechuan Veggie Dumpling Soup (page 114).

1. Boil the edamame according to package directions. Drain, rinse with cold water, and drain again. Add the edamame, hoisin sauce, sesame oil, soy sauce, and hot pepper flakes to a food processor. Cover and blend until the mixture forms a thick, smooth paste, scraping down the sides as needed. Transfer to a medium bowl and stir in the scallions, ginger, garlic, and cilantro until combined.

2. One at a time, brush the edges of each wrapper with fresh, cold water. Place 2 teaspoons edamame mixture in the center of the wrapper. Fold one side of the wrapper over the filling to form a half moon, and pinch the edges. Crimp the edges with fork tongs, if desired. Keep the dumplings covered with a damp, clean kitchen towel.

3. Preheat the oven to 200°F. Bring about 1 inch of water to a simmer over medium heat. Spritz a

steamer basket with cooking spray to help prevent sticking before each batch. Place 8 dumplings (or as many dumplings as can fit) into the steamer without them touching. Cover and steam until the dumplings are cooked through, about 10 minutes. Remove the dumplings from the steamer to a heatproof platter and place in the oven to keep warm. (Spritz the dumplings with cooking spray, if necessary, to prevent sticking and keep them moist.) Repeat until all of the dumplings are steamed, adding additional water for simmering between batches, if necessary.

4. Transfer the dumplings to a platter or individual plates and garnish with additional minced scallions (green parts), if desired. Enjoy the dumplings while warm.

{ WITH POULTRY, FISH, OR MEAT }

One serving: Mince 1-ounce fresh, wild, dry sea scallops or boneless, skinless chicken breast. Stir it into 2 tablespoons edamame filling for the last 3 dumpling wrappers you plan to fill in step 2. Use one more dumpling wrapper, creating 4 dumplings for the serving, since there is more filling to work with. Prepare these as a final batch in step 3.

Full recipe: Mince 8 ounces fresh, wild, dry sea scallops or boneless, skinless chicken breast. Stir into the edamame filling at the end of step 1. Use 32 instead of 24 dumpling wrappers, creating 4 dumplings for each serving.

without
Exchanges/Food Choices: 1 Starch, 1/2 Fat
80 calories, 20 calories from fat, 2.5g total fat, 0g saturated fat, 0g trans fat, 0mg cholesterol, 140mg sodium, 160mg potassium, 12g total carbohydrate, 1g dietary fiber, 2g sugars, 4g protein, 60mg phosphorus

with
Exchanges/Food Choices: 1 Starch, 1 Lean Meat
130 calories, 25 calories from fat, 2.5g total fat, 0g saturated fat, 0g trans fat, 10mg cholesterol, 320mg sodium, 250mg potassium, 17g total carbohydrate, 1g dietary fiber, 2g sugars, 10g protein, 200mg phosphorus

Grilled Figs with Balsamic Reduction

Makes 4 servings: 3 fig halves each

1/4 cup aged (8–10 years) balsamic vinegar

6 fresh Black Mission or Striped Tiger figs, stemmed, halved lengthwise

Cooking spray

1/8 teaspoon sea salt, or to taste

1 tablespoon lightly salted roasted pistachios, chopped

1 teaspoon chopped fresh rosemary leaves

1/4 teaspoon freshly ground black pepper, or to taste

I adore fresh figs of late summer. I often eat most of them before I gather up ingredients to use them in a recipe. Here's a recipe that I'm sure to save six nicely sized fig beauties for, though. Be sure to do the same. Grilling the figs creates enticing caramelization. Finishing with a drizzling of a deep and distinctive balsamic vinegar reduction and a sprinkling of crunchy pistachios, this sweet and savory appetizer will have amazing appeal for your palate.

1. Bring the vinegar to a boil in a small saucepan over high heat. Reduce heat to medium-low and simmer until the vinegar reduces by about half, about 7 minutes. Set aside to cool.

2. Prepare an outdoor or indoor grill or grill pan. Spritz the cut surface of each fig half with cooking spray. Grill over direct medium-high heat on the cut side until caramelized, about 3 1/2 minutes.

3. Arrange the fig halves on a platter. Sprinkle with the salt and drizzle with desired amount of the balsamic reduction. Sprinkle with the pistachios, rosemary, and pepper. Serve at room temperature.

One serving: Cut a 1/2-ounce extra-thin slice of prosciutto or American country ham into thirds lengthwise. Wrap one piece around each of 3 grilled fig halves before arranging on a platter in step 3. Do not add salt. Serve on a separate plate.

Full recipe: Cut four 1/2-ounce extra-thin slices of prosciutto or American country ham into thirds lengthwise. Wrap one piece around each grilled fig half before arranging on a platter in step 3. Do not add salt.

without
Exchanges/Food Choices: 1/2 Fruit,
1/2 Carbohydrate
80 calories, 15 calories from fat, 1.5g total fat,
0g saturated fat, 0g trans fat, 0mg cholesterol,
85mg sodium, 210mg potassium, 18g total
carbohydrate, 2g dietary fiber, 15g sugars,
1g protein, 20mg phosphorus

with
Exchanges/Food Choices: 1/2 Fruit,
1/2 Carbohydrate, 1 Lean Meat, 1/2 Fat
120 calories, 25 calories from fat, 3g total fat,
0.5g saturated fat, 0g trans fat, 10mg cholesterol,
390mg sodium, 290mg potassium, 18g total
carbohydrate, 2g dietary fiber, 15g sugars,
5g protein, 70mg phosphorus

Do-It-Yourself Cooking Spray

Cooking spray enables you to spritz just a tiny amount of oil onto foods. But rather than buying an aerosol can cooking spray, I suggest filling a spray bottle, like a Misto Gourmet Sprayer, with your desired cooking oil… and nothing else. You can select the oil that best matches your recipe, taste preferences, or health needs—or all of the above. I often choose extra-virgin olive oil, though grapeseed oil will be more versatile.

Baby Bella Blue Nachos

Makes 6 servings: 4 nachos each

1/2 cup plain fat-free Greek yogurt

1 teaspoon fresh lime juice, or to taste

2 teaspoons canola or grapeseed oil

2 scallions, thinly sliced, green and white parts separated

4 cups thinly sliced or chopped crimini (baby bella) mushrooms (10 ounces)

1/4 teaspoon chili powder, or to taste

1/4 teaspoon sea salt, or to taste

1/4 cup thick "hot" or medium salsa

24 large blue or yellow corn tortilla chips

1 cup shredded vegan Monterey Jack cheese alternative (4 ounces) or 3/4 cup shredded Monterey Jack cheese (3 ounces)

24 fresh cilantro leaves

12 grape tomatoes or small cherry tomatoes, cut in half lengthwise

Nachos are not considered to be upscale or healthful. That's all changed now. Get a load of these bodacious baby bella–spiked nachos. Each blue tortilla chip is topped individually, so its scrumptiousness can be savored slowly. These nachos will fill your cheese craving, but consider using a vegan cheese alternative so they're as plant-based as possible. Using a spicy salsa gives zing, and a lime-accented Greek yogurt creates an extra-creamy finish. Now there's no need to say "no" to nachos.

1. Combine the yogurt and lime juice in a small bowl, and set aside.

2. Heat the oil in a large, nonstick skillet over medium-high heat. Add the white part of the scallions, the mushrooms, chili powder, and salt, and sauté until the mushrooms are just cooked through, about 5 minutes. Stir in the salsa and the green part of the scallions, and sauté until no excess liquid remains, about 5 minutes more.

3. Arrange the tortilla chips on small, microwave-safe plates, 4 chips each. Top each chip with about 1 tablespoon mushroom mixture and a pinch of the cheese. Microwave each serving on high until the cheese is just melted, about 30 seconds.

4. Top each nacho with 1 teaspoon yogurt mixture, a cilantro leaf, and a grape tomato half. Serve while warm.

{ WITH POULTRY, FISH, OR MEAT }

One serving: Dice 1 ounce rotisserie or roasted chicken breast meat. Top 4 tortilla chips with the chicken and a pinch of ground cumin and freshly ground black pepper before adding the cheese in step 3.

Full recipe: Dice 6 ounces rotisserie or roasted chicken breast meat and season with 1/4 teaspoon ground cumin and 1/4 teaspoon freshly ground black pepper. Top the tortilla chips with the chicken before adding the cheese in step 3.

without
Exchanges/Food Choices: 1/2 Starch,
1 Vegetable, 1 1/2 Fat
150 calories, 80 calories from fat, 9g total fat,
1g saturated fat, 0g trans fat, 0mg cholesterol,
300mg sodium, 310mg potassium, 13g total
carbohydrate, 2g dietary fiber, 3g sugars,
5g protein, 90mg phosphorus

with
Exchanges/Food Choices: 1/2 Starch,
1 Vegetable, 1 Lean Meat, 1 1/2 Fat
190 calories, 90 calories from fat, 10g total fat,
1g saturated fat, 0g trans fat, 25mg cholesterol,
390mg sodium, 400mg potassium, 13g total
carbohydrate, 2g dietary fiber, 3g sugars,
13g protein, 160mg phosphorus

Herb and Spice Tofu Salad "Bruschetta"

Makes 6 servings: 2 "bruschetta" each

2 scallions, green and white parts, minced

3 tablespoons mayonnaise or vegan mayonnaise

1 1/2 tablespoons whole-grain mustard

1 1/2 tablespoons finely chopped fresh flat-leaf parsley

1 tablespoon finely chopped fresh tarragon

1/2 teaspoon ground cayenne pepper, or to taste

1/4 teaspoon ground turmeric

1/4 teaspoon + 1/8 teaspoon sea salt, or to taste

1/4 teaspoon freshly ground black pepper, or to taste

1 medium celery stalk, finely diced

1 (14-ounce) package firm tofu, drained and squeezed of excess liquid

12 slices light rye crispbread

Here's one of my preferred ways to savor tofu as a snack. The spices create notable kick, and the herbs provide aromatic goodness. There's nothing glamorous about it, but sometimes it's just about grabbing good grub, not pretty bites. The tofu topping looks like egg salad, but you'll likely find it more appetizing. I use light rye crispbread that is just 30 calories a slice to keep this calorie-friendly but provide great crunch and satisfaction. I hope you find this interesting "bruschetta" as delightful and delicious as I do.

1. Stir together the scallions, mayonnaise, mustard, parsley, tarragon, cayenne, turmeric, salt, and pepper in a medium bowl until well combined. Add the celery, and stir until evenly combined.

2. Mash the tofu in a large bowl using a large spoon until small, bite-size crumbles are formed.

3. Stir the tofu into the celery mixture. Chill for at least 1 hour to let flavors blend. Adjust seasoning.

4. Top each crispbread with about 3 tablespoons tofu mixture, and serve.

{ WITH POULTRY, FISH, OR MEAT }

One serving: Transfer 1 rounded tablespoon celery mixture to a small bowl at the end of step 1. Mash about 12 ounces tofu (instead of the 14 ounces) in a large bowl in step 2. Stir the tofu into the celery mixture in the medium bowl. Then, stir 2 ounces flaked, water-packed, canned, no-salt-added white, low-mercury Albacore tuna, or chilled, shredded, roasted chicken thigh, into the celery mixture in the small bowl. Do not drain the tuna.

Full recipe: Replace the tofu in the recipe with 12 ounces flaked, water-packed, canned, no-salt-added white, low-mercury Albacore tuna, or chilled, shredded, roasted chicken thigh. Do not drain the tuna.

without
Exchanges/Food Choices: 1 Starch, 1 Lean Meat, 1 Fat
170 calories, 80 calories from fat, 9g total fat, 1.5g saturated fat, 0g trans fat, 5mg cholesterol, 360mg sodium, 200mg potassium, 16g total carbohydrate, 4g dietary fiber, 1g sugars, 7g protein, 130mg phosphorus

with
Exchanges/Food Choices: 1 Starch, 2 Lean Meat, 1/2 Fat
190 calories, 70 calories from fat, 7g total fat, 1g saturated fat, 0g trans fat, 25mg cholesterol, 380mg sodium, 230mg potassium, 15g total carbohydrate, 3g dietary fiber, 0g sugars, 15g protein, 170mg phosphorus

Hummus, Avocado, and Tomato Rounds

Makes 4 servings: 1 topped toasted muffin each

2 medium vine-ripened tomatoes or Kumato tomatoes, halved lengthwise, cores and seeds removed

Olive oil cooking spray

1 1/2 teaspoons fresh lemon juice, divided

1/8 teaspoon sea salt, divided

1 Hass avocado, pitted and peeled

2 whole-grain English muffins, split

1/3 cup hummus of choice (page 59)

1 teaspoon finely chopped fresh basil

1/8 teaspoon freshly ground black pepper, or to taste

1 tablespoon unsalted roasted pistachios, chopped, or toasted pine nuts (optional)

Need a show-stopping appetizer to impress guests or dazzle your family? This is it! It's kind of like a glammed up open-face sandwich. A toasted English muffin is generously topped with layers of creamy hummus, fresh avocado, and roasted tomato. Try it with the unique and intense-tasting Kumato tomatoes, which are considered brown tomatoes, for an interesting taste and color twist.

1. Preheat the oven to 425°F. Arrange the tomatoes cut side up on an 8-inch square baking pan lined with unbleached parchment paper. Spritz the tomatoes with olive oil cooking spray and sprinkle with 1/2 teaspoon lemon juice and a pinch of salt. Roast until the tomatoes are caramelized, about 45 minutes. Let stand for at least 5 minutes.

2. Meanwhile, gently mash the avocado with the remaining 1 teaspoon lemon juice and a pinch of salt in a medium bowl. Adjust seasoning.

3. Toast the 4 English muffin halves. Spread each with hummus. Layer the mashed avocado over the hummus. Top each muffin with a roasted tomato, sprinkle with the basil, pepper, and pistachios (if using), and serve.

One serving: Transfer 1/4 of the avocado mixture in step 2 to a small bowl and stir 3/4 ounce finely cubed roasted, or rotisserie, chicken breast meat into this mixture. Spread atop the hummus of one of the English muffin halves in step 3.

Full recipe: Stir 3 ounces finely cubed roasted, or rotisserie, chicken breast meat into the avocado mixture in step 2.

without
Exchanges/Food Choices: 1 Starch, 1 Vegetable, 1 Fat
170 calories, 70 calories from fat, 8g total fat, 1g saturated fat, 0g trans fat, 0mg cholesterol, 270mg sodium, 440mg potassium, 22g total carbohydrate, 6g dietary fiber, 4g sugars, 6g protein, 162mg phosphorus

with
Exchanges/Food Choices: 1 Starch, 1 Vegetable, 1 Lean Meat, 1 Fat
200 calories, 80 calories from fat, 9g total fat, 1.4g saturated fat, 0g trans fat, 20mg cholesterol, 290mg sodium, 490mg potassium, 22g total carbohydrate, 6g dietary fiber, 4g sugars, 12g protein, 210mg phosphorus

Hummus

Some recipes suggest using "hummus of choice." You can use your favorite store-bought variety, your own recipe, or mine:

Jackie's Classic Hummus

Makes 14 servings: 2 tablespoons each

1 (15-ounce) can no-salt-added chickpeas (garbanzo beans), drained
1/4 cup tahini
1/4 cup unsweetened green tea, chilled
Juice of 1 small lemon (2 tablespoons)

1 large garlic clove, chopped
1/2 teaspoon sea salt
1/4 teaspoon ground cumin
1/8 teaspoon ground cayenne pepper (optional)

Add all of the ingredients to a food processor or blender. Cover, purée, and serve. Makes 1 3/4 cups.

Exchanges/Food Choices: 1/2 Starch, 1/2 Fat
60 calories, 25 calories from fat, 2.5g total fat, 0g saturated fat, 0g trans fat, 0mg cholesterol, 90mg sodium, 80mg potassium, 7g total carbohydrate, 1g dietary fiber, 0g sugars, 2g protein, 60mg phosphorus

Pizzette al Funghi

2 cups sliced mushroom mixture

2 teaspoons extra-virgin olive oil

2 large garlic cloves, minced

2 tablespoons minced fresh chives

1 teaspoon finely chopped fresh rosemary

1/4 teaspoon freshly ground black pepper, or to taste

1/8 teaspoon sea salt, or to taste

2 (2-ounce) whole-grain soft thin flatbreads

1/3 cup finely crumbled soft goat cheese, at room temperature (1.5 ounces)

6 large sun-dried tomatoes (not oil-packed), thinly sliced, rehydrated

1/4 cup shredded vegan mozzarella cheese alternative or part-skim mozzarella cheese (1 ounce)

1/8 teaspoon dried hot pepper flakes, or to taste

2 tablespoons roughly chopped fresh flat-leaf parsley

Yes, pizza can be part of your meal repertoire…regularly! Here, using a thin crust is part of the trick to helping it fit into a healthy eating plan. Then, playing with a variety of plant-based toppings creates cuisine drama. Sun-dried tomatoes provide more flavor-pep than pepperoni. Mushrooms (a.k.a. funghi) are captivating and make each piece of pizzette especially satiating. Use an interesting mixture, like oyster, maitake, and beech mushrooms. The herbs and spice make it extra nice.

1. Preheat the oven to 450°F. Toss the mushrooms with the oil, garlic, chives, rosemary, black pepper, and salt in a medium bowl.

2. Sprinkle the entire surface of each flatbread with the goat cheese. Top with the mushroom mixture, sun-dried tomatoes, mozzarella cheese alternative, and hot pepper flakes.

3. Place both pizzettes on a large baking sheet and bake until the crust is browned and crisp, about 12 minutes. Remove from the oven. Adjust seasoning.

4. Cut each pizzette into quarters with a pizza cutter. Arrange pieces on a platter, sprinkle with the parsley, and serve immediately.

{ WITH POULTRY, FISH, OR MEAT }

One serving: Before topping the flatbreads with the sun-dried tomatoes in step 2, top one-quarter of one of the flatbreads with thin slices ("coins") from 1/2 ounce precooked Italian poultry sausage link. Do not heat sausage before use.

Full recipe: Before topping the flatbreads with the sun-dried tomatoes in step 2, top with thin slices ("coins") from 4 ounces precooked Italian poultry sausage links. Do not heat sausage before use.

without
Exchanges/Food Choices: 1/2 Starch, 1 Fat
80 calories, 35 calories from fat, 3.5g total fat,
1g saturated fat, 0g trans fat, 0mg cholesterol,
140mg sodium, 160mg potassium, 10g total
carbohydrate, 2g dietary fiber, 1g sugars,
3g protein, 70mg phosphorus

with
Exchanges/Food Choices: 1/2 Starch,1 Fat
100 calories, 45 calories from fat, 5g total fat,
1.5g saturated fat, 0g trans fat, 10mg cholesterol,
270mg sodium, 190mg potassium, 11g total
carbohydrate, 2g dietary fiber, 1g sugars,
6g protein, 90mg phosphorus

Sea Salt and White Asparagus Pizza Crisps

Makes 8 servings: 1 wedge each

2 large (10-inch) whole-wheat tortillas or wraps

Olive oil cooking spray

1/2 cup shredded part-skim mozzarella cheese (2 ounces)

8 steamed white asparagus stalks, chilled, sliced into 1/4-inch or thinner "coins," ends trimmed

1/4 teaspoon sea salt, preferably flaked, or to taste

1/4 cup sun-dried tomatoes, rehydrated, thinly sliced

1 shallot, very thinly sliced

2 teaspoons grated Pecorino Romano or Parmigiano-Reggiano cheese

1 teaspoon finely chopped fresh rosemary

1/4 teaspoon freshly ground black pepper, or to taste

Pizza isn't junk food, especially when generously topped with veggies. Here, the pizza crust is extra thin and crispy, so the pizza will seem cheesier than expected. The toppings are the focus, and the main highlight is the white asparagus, which gives it an elegant touch. Even sea salt is a distinctive ingredient here. This is definitely no ordinary slice.

1. Preheat the oven to 400°F. Lightly coat both sides of the tortillas with olive oil cooking spray. Place the tortillas on an oven-safe rack placed on a large baking sheet or directly onto an extra-large perforated pizza pan. In order, top the entire surface of both tortillas with the mozzarella cheese, asparagus, salt, sun-dried tomatoes, and the shallot. Spritz with cooking spray. Sprinkle with the Romano cheese, rosemary, and pepper.

2. Bake until the tortillas are crisp and brown, mozzarella is melted, and asparagus is fully roasted, about 25 minutes.

3. Cut into 4 wedges each, and serve immediately. If not serving immediately, keep the pizzas on the rack to help maintain crispness, and serve at room temperature.

{ WITH POULTRY, FISH, OR MEAT }

One serving: Slice about 0.4 ounce precooked Italian poultry sausage link into extra-thin "coins." Sprinkle onto 1/4 of one of the pizzas before the mozzarella cheese in step 1. Do not heat sausage before use.

Full recipe: Slice a 3-ounce precooked Italian poultry sausage link into extra-thin "coins." Sprinkle onto the pizzas before the mozzarella cheese in step 1. Do not heat sausage before use.

without
Exchanges/Food Choices: 1/2 Starch, 1 Vegetable, 1/2 Fat
90 calories, 20 calories from fat, 2.5g total fat, 1g saturated fat, 0g trans fat, 5mg cholesterol, 260mg sodium, 210mg potassium, 13g total carbohydrate, 2g dietary fiber, 3g sugars, 4g protein, 90mg phosphorus

with
Exchanges/Food Choices: 1/2 Starch, 1 Vegetable, 1 Medium-Fat Meat
110 calories, 30 calories from fat, 3.5g total fat, 1.5g saturated fat, 0g trans fat, 10mg cholesterol, 360mg sodium, 230mg potassium, 13g total carbohydrate, 2g dietary fiber, 3g sugars, 6g protein, 110mg phosphorus

Peach and Black Bean Salsa with Chips

Makes 8 servings: 1/3 rounded cup salsa with 6 chips each

Juice of 1 lime (2 tablespoons)

1 small jalapeño pepper, with some seeds, minced

1/4 teaspoon sea salt, or to taste

1/4 teaspoon freshly ground black pepper

1 tablespoon unrefined peanut or flaxseed oil

1 large fresh peach, pitted and finely diced

3 scallions, green and white parts, thinly sliced

1/2 teaspoon finely chopped fresh oregano leaves

1 (15-ounce) can black beans, gently rinsed and drained (1 1/2 cups)

48 blue corn or sweet potato tortilla chips

Salsa usually refers to a tomato-based, sometimes spicy sauce that's served dip-style with tortilla chips. Here, however, the tried and true gets a new twist. Instead of tomato, there's juicy peach. (Hint: Use a fully ripened peach so that it's lusciously sweet tasting.) To balance it out and give it great body, I've incorporated black beans. Now this lively salsa, with its Caribbean accent, can be served as a satisfying salad, not just as a dip for chips.

1. Add the lime juice, jalapeño, salt, and pepper to a medium bowl. Whisk in the oil until well combined. Stir in the peach, scallions, and oregano until combined. Stir in the beans and adjust seasoning.

2. Arrange the tortilla chips on a platter around a bowl of the salsa, and serve at room temperature. Alternatively, serve individual portions of salsa with the chips.

WITH POULTRY, FISH, OR MEAT

One serving: After stirring in the beans in step 1, transfer 1/3 rounded cup peach and bean salsa to a small bowl. Stir 2 ounces picked-over, premium, wild claw lump crabmeat chunks into the mixture in the small bowl. Adjust seasoning.

Full recipe: Stir 1 pound picked-over, premium, wild claw lump crabmeat chunks into the peach and bean salsa in step 1. Adjust seasoning.

without
Exchanges/Food Choices: 1 1/2 Starch, 1 Fat
150 calories, 50 calories from fat,
6g total fat, 1g saturated fat, 0g trans fat,
0mg cholesterol, 180mg sodium,
200mg potassium, 22g total carbohydrate,
3g dietary fiber, 4g sugars, 4g protein,
90mg phosphorus

with
Exchanges/Food Choices: 1 1/2 Starch,
2 Lean Meat, 1 Fat
200 calories, 50 calories from fat,
6g total fat, 1g saturated fat, 0g trans fat,
55mg cholesterol, 410mg sodium,
350mg potassium, 22g total carbohydrate,
3g dietary fiber, 4g sugars, 14g protein,
230mg phosphorus

CHAPTER 3

salads

All-American Broccoli Slaw

Makes 6 servings: about 1 cup each

3/4 cup plain fat-free yogurt (6 ounces)

2 tablespoons no-sugar-added apple-peach sauce or applesauce

2 tablespoons apple cider vinegar, or to taste

1/4 teaspoon sea salt, or to taste

1 (12-ounce) bag broccoli slaw

1 small red onion, finely diced

1/2 cup black seedless raisins or finely chopped dried unsulphured apricots

1/3 cup dry-roasted lightly salted peanuts

without
Exchanges/Food Choices: 1 Fruit, 1 Vegetable, 1 Fat
140 calories, 40 calories from fat, 4.5g total fat, 1g saturated fat, 0g trans fat, 0mg cholesterol, 170mg sodium, 440mg potassium, 21g total carbohydrate, 3g dietary fiber, 13g sugars, 6g protein, 130mg phosphorus

with
Exchanges/Food Choices: 1 Fruit, 1 Vegetable, 1 1/2 Fat
170 calories, 50 calories from fat, 6g total fat, 1g saturated fat, 0g trans fat, 25mg cholesterol, 370mg sodium, 480mg potassium, 21g total carbohydrate, 3g dietary fiber, 13g sugars, 12g protein, 170mg phosphorus

Slaws don't always need to be made with cabbage. Broccoli provides an excellent, family-friendly alternative. Plus, you can cheat and buy a bag already shredded into slaw. Otherwise, try a 4-cup packed mixture of shredded broccoli, carrots, and red cabbage. The dressing is sweetened naturally with fruit sauce and is mayo-free. The combination of yogurt and cider vinegar provides a creamy tang so the mayo won't be missed. Finished with a generous sprinkling of raisins and peanuts, there's something in this slaw that every one of your taste buds will fancy.

1. Whisk together the yogurt, apple-peach sauce, vinegar, and salt in a large bowl. Add the broccoli slaw, onion, and raisins, and toss to combine.

2. Let stand for 30 minutes to allow flavors to blend. Toss again, and adjust seasoning.

3. Sprinkle with the peanuts, and serve.

WITH POULTRY, FISH, OR MEAT

One serving: Transfer 1 cup slaw to a small bowl when ready to serve in step 3. Finely chop 1 slice of cooked, hardwood-smoked, uncured turkey bacon or Sunday bacon and toss into the slaw.

Full recipe: Finely chop 6 slices of cooked, hardwood-smoked, uncured turkey bacon or Sunday bacon and toss into the slaw before sprinkling with the peanuts in step 3.

Asian Herb and Almond Savoy Slaw

Makes 6 servings: 1 cup each

Consider this recipe coleslaw gone global. The basil and the cilantro finish it with fresh fragrance, the almonds with nutty crunch. It's an enticing pick for picnics or other gatherings. Just toss the veggies and prepare the sauce separately. Then combine veggies with the sauce when ready to serve. The full-flavored slaw will add Asian flair to any meal.

1. Whisk together the vinegar, apple-peach sauce, almond butter, soy sauce, mustard, sesame oil, ginger, and garlic-chili sauce in a medium bowl.

2. Toss together the cabbage, bell pepper, scallions, and basil in a large bowl.

3. When ready to serve, add the sauce mixture to the cabbage mixture and toss to coat.

4. Transfer to a platter, sprinkle with the almonds, and serve.

WITH POULTRY, FISH, OR MEAT

One serving: After tossing together the cabbage and sauce mixture in step 3, transfer 1 cup slaw to a small bowl. Add 1 1/2 ounces thin strips of grilled or roasted chicken breast to the slaw and toss to combine. Sprinkle with 2 teaspoons almonds.

Full recipe: Stir 9 ounces thin strips of grilled or roasted chicken breast into the sauce at the end of step 1.

2 tablespoons brown rice vinegar

2 tablespoons no-sugar-added apple-peach sauce or applesauce

2 tablespoons roasted no-salt-added creamy almond butter

1 tablespoon naturally brewed soy sauce

1 tablespoon whole-grain mustard

2 teaspoons toasted sesame oil

2 teaspoons freshly grated gingerroot

1 teaspoon Asian garlic-chili sauce

6 cups packed shredded Savoy cabbage (1/2 head)

1 medium orange bell pepper, very thinly sliced into 2-inch strips

3 scallions, green and white parts, thinly sliced on the diagonal

1/3 cup finely chopped fresh basil or mixture of basil and cilantro

1/4 cup sliced natural almonds, toasted

without

Exchanges/Food Choices: 1 Vegetable, 1 1/2 Fat
100 calories, 60 calories from fat, 7g total fat, 0.5g saturated fat, 0g trans fat, 0mg cholesterol, 240mg sodium, 270mg potassium, 9g total carbohydrate, 3g dietary fiber, 4g sugars, 4g protein, 80mg phosphorus

with

Exchanges/Food Choices: 1 Vegetable, 1 1/2 Lean Meat, 1 1/2 Fat
170 calories, 70 calories from fat, 8g total fat, 1g saturated fat, 0g trans fat, 35mg cholesterol, 270mg sodium, 380mg potassium, 9g total carbohydrate, 3g dietary fiber, 4g sugars, 17g protein, 180mg phosphorus

Peppercorn Pistachio Caesar-Style Salad

Makes 4 servings: 2 cups each

1 large sweet potato, unpeeled, cut into 12 slices crosswise

2 teaspoons canola or roasted pistachio oil

1/3 cup hummus of choice (page 59)

3 tablespoons unsweetened green tea, chilled

3 tablespoons grated Parmigiano-Reggiano cheese

2 large garlic cloves

1 tablespoon Dijon mustard

2 teaspoons vegetarian Worcestershire sauce

2 teaspoons lemon juice

1 1/4 teaspoons freshly cracked black peppercorns, or to taste, divided

8 cups packed field greens or mesclun salad (8 ounces)

2 tablespoons chopped, lightly salted, roasted shelled pistachios

Here's a Caesar-inspired salad that's filled with intrigue. The dressing is cleverly based on hummus and green tea. The combination of Dijon mustard, vegetarian Worcestershire sauce, and plenty of pepper allows the dressing to go anchovy-free and also provides lots of distinctive taste. Grilled sweet potato rounds make the salad more substantial and attention-grabbing. Finally, pistachios provide crunch better than croutons ever could. This salad is every bit the tempter.

1. Preheat a grill or grill pan. Brush the sweet potato slices with the oil. Grill over direct medium heat until fully cooked and grill marks form, about 8 minutes per side. Set aside.

2. Add the hummus, tea, cheese, garlic, mustard, Worcestershire sauce, lemon juice, and 1 teaspoon peppercorns to a blender. Cover and purée.

3. When ready to serve, toss the dressing with the greens in a large mixing bowl. Transfer to 4 separate bowls or plates, top with the grilled sweet potato slices, sprinkle with the pistachios and the remaining 1/4 teaspoon peppercorns, and serve.

{ WITH POULTRY, FISH, OR MEAT }

One serving: Use a medium instead of large sweet potato for step 1; slice into 9 "coins" and brush with 1 1/2 teaspoons oil. After grilling the sweet potato slices, brush 3 ounces wild Atlantic salmon or boneless, skinless chicken thigh with the remaining 1/2 teaspoon oil and grill until done; add a pinch of sea salt. In step 3, top 3 salads with the sweet potato slices and the fourth with the salmon, whole or flaked.

Full recipe: Instead of the sweet potato in step 1, grill four 3-ounce portions of wild Atlantic salmon or boneless, skinless chicken thigh; add 1/4 teaspoon sea salt. In step 3, top each salad with the salmon, whole or flaked, before sprinkling with the pistachios.

without
Exchanges/Food Choices: 1 Carbohydrate,
1 Vegetable, 1 1/2 Fat
160 calories, 70 calories from fat, 7g total fat,
1.5g saturated fat, 0g trans fat,
5mg cholesterol, 340mg sodium,
440mg potassium, 20g total carbohydrate,
5g dietary fiber, 4g sugars, 6g protein,
120mg phosphorus

with
Exchanges/Food Choices: 1/2 Carbohydrate,
1 Vegetable, 3 Lean Meat, 1 1/2 Fat
260 calories, 120 calories from fat, 13g total
fat, 2.5g saturated fat, 0g trans fat,
55mg cholesterol, 510mg sodium,
700mg potassium, 11g total carbohydrate,
4g dietary fiber, 1g sugars, 25g protein,
290mg phosphorus

Grilled Spring Asparagus Salad

Makes 4 servings: 1 1/2 cups salad with 6 asparagus spears each

24 asparagus spears, ends trimmed

1 1/2 tablespoon extra-virgin olive oil, divided

1/8 teaspoon sea salt (optional)

Juice of 1 small lemon (2 tablespoons)

6 cups packed mesclun or mixed baby salad greens (6 ounces)

2 tablespoons thinly sliced fresh basil

1/3 cup minced red onion, divided

1/4 teaspoon freshly ground black pepper, or to taste

without
Exchanges/Food Choices: 2 Vegetable, 1 Fat
80 calories, 50 calories from fat, 6g total fat, 1g saturated fat, 0g trans fat, 0mg cholesterol, 35mg sodium, 430mg potassium, 7g total carbohydrate, 3g dietary fiber, 2g sugars, 4g protein, 80mg phosphorus

with
Exchanges/Food Choices: 2 Vegetable, 1 1/2 Fat
110 calories, 60 calories from fat, 7g total fat, 1g saturated fat, 0g trans fat, 10mg cholesterol, 420mg sodium, 500mg potassium, 7g total carbohydrate, 3g dietary fiber, 2g sugars, 7g protein, 120mg phosphorus

Grilled asparagus seems downright addictive to me. I indulge on spears like French fries ... no ketchup, of course! Here they transform a simple salad into one that's wow-worthy. The lemony vinaigrette brings it all together in perfect culinary harmony. If you pick up the asparagus spears from this salad with your fingers, I promise I won't tell anyone! Using a fork and a knife is more polite, of course.

1. Prepare an outdoor or indoor grill. Place the asparagus into a 9 × 13-inch dish, sprinkle with 1/2 tablespoon oil and the salt (if using), and toss to coat.

2. Grill the asparagus (in batches, if necessary) until lightly charred and just tender over medium-high heat, turning only as needed, about 8–10 minutes.

3. Meanwhile, whisk together the lemon juice with the remaining 1 tablespoon oil in a large bowl. Add the mesclun, basil, and half of the onion, and toss to coat. Arrange the mesclun salad on individual plates.

4. Top each salad with 6 grilled asparagus spears. Sprinkle with the remaining onion and the pepper, and serve.

WITH POULTRY, FISH, OR MEAT

One serving: Wrap a 1/2-ounce extra-thin slice of prosciutto or American country ham around one set of 6 asparagus spears and arrange on one of the salads in step 4.

Full recipe: Wrap a 1/2-ounce extra-thin slice of prosciutto or American country ham around each set of 6 asparagus spears and arrange on each salad in step 4.

Hominy Taco Salad

Makes 4 servings: about 2 cups each

I introduced salad to a tortilla chip snack to create this harmonious result. The dressing has a definite tang to it, which works magically to balance all of the other flavors of this crunchy salad. The hominy makes it a standout, though you can use yellow corn in its place. It's a salad that the whole family will love.

1. Add the yogurt, cilantro, lime juice, and oil to a blender. Cover and purée.
2. Toss together the baby greens, hominy, tomatoes, bell pepper, jalapeño, and the cilantro-yogurt dressing in a large bowl.
3. Arrange the salad onto 4 plates, sprinkle with the black pepper, garnish with the chips, and serve.

{ WITH POULTRY, FISH, OR MEAT }

One serving: Season a 2-ounce piece of well-trimmed, boneless, grass-fed New York strip or sirloin steak with a smidgen each of sea salt and freshly ground black pepper. Grill or pan-grill over direct medium-high heat until desired doneness, about 3 minutes per side for medium-rare. Let stand for at least 5 minutes to complete the cooking process. Thinly slice against the grain, then arrange onto one of the salads in step 3 before sprinkling with the black pepper from the main recipe.

Full recipe: Season 8 ounces well-trimmed, boneless, grass-fed New York strip or sirloin steak, about 1 1/4 inches thick, with 1/8 teaspoon each sea salt and freshly ground black pepper. Grill or pan-grill over direct medium-high heat until desired doneness, about 3 1/2 minutes per side for medium-rare. Let stand for at least 5 minutes to complete the cooking process. Thinly slice against the grain, then arrange onto the salads in step 3 before sprinkling with the black pepper from the main recipe.

1/3 cup plain fat-free yogurt

1/4 cup fresh cilantro leaves

Juice of 1/2 lime (1 tablespoon)

1 tablespoon extra-virgin olive oil

5 cups packed fresh baby greens (5 ounces)

1 1/2 cups cooked white hominy, chilled, or 1 (15-ounce) can drained white hominy (posole)

12 cherry or large grape tomatoes, quartered, drained of excess liquids

1 medium green bell pepper, diced

1 small jalapeño pepper, with some seeds, halved lengthwise and thinly sliced crosswise

1/2 teaspoon freshly ground black pepper, or to taste

16 blue or yellow corn tortilla chips

without
Exchanges/Food Choices: 1 1/2 Starch, 1 Vegetable, 1 Fat
180 calories, 60 calories from fat, 6g total fat, 1g saturated fat, 0g trans fat, 0mg cholesterol, 420mg sodium, 360mg potassium, 27g total carbohydrate, 5g dietary fiber, 6g sugars, 4g protein, 90mg phosphorus

with
Exchanges/Food Choices: 1 1/2 Starch, 1 Vegetable, 2 Lean Meat, 1 Fat
250 calories, 70 calories from fat, 8g total fat, 1.5g saturated fat, 0g trans fat, 30mg cholesterol, 540mg sodium, 460mg potassium, 28g total carbohydrate, 6g dietary fiber, 6g sugars, 17g protein, 200mg phosphorus

Fresh Mint and Baby Spinach Salad with Grapes

Makes 4 servings: 2 1/2 cups each

Juice and zest of 1 small lemon
(2 tablespoons juice)

1 tablespoon extra-virgin olive oil

1/4 teaspoon sea salt, or to taste

1/2 teaspoon freshly ground black
pepper, divided

1 1/3 cups seedless red grapes,
halved lengthwise, divided

5 cups packed fresh baby spinach
(5 ounces)

2 (5-ounce) Kirby cucumbers or
10 ounces English cucumber,
unpeeled, halved lengthwise and
thinly sliced crosswise

1/2 cup packed fresh small whole
mint leaves

1/3 cup extra-thinly sliced red onion

2 tablespoons pine nuts, toasted

Can you smell the mint yet? So refreshing! This salad hits all of the right notes when you want a leafy salad that's fresh, fragrant, fruity, and flavorful. It's actually a recipe that I put together with extra ingredients I happened to have on hand one day, and it's become one of my all-time favorites. The salad is dressed with a fresh grape vinaigrette that's delightful. It has feminine appeal, but I dare the guys to dig into this. Think of it like an equal-opportunity palate pleaser.

1. Add the lemon juice, oil, salt, 1/4 teaspoon pepper, and 1/3 cup grapes to a blender. Cover and purée. (Note: Tiny flecks from the grape skins will remain.) Set aside.

2. Toss together the spinach, cucumbers, mint, and onion in a large bowl.

3. Drizzle the vinaigrette over the salad and toss to coat.

4. Transfer the salad to 4 individual plates or a large platter. Sprinkle with remaining 1 cup grapes, the pine nuts, desired amount of the lemon zest, and the remaining 1/4 teaspoon pepper. Adjust seasoning, and serve.

{ WITH POULTRY, FISH, OR MEAT }

One serving: Transfer about 2 cups dressed salad at the end of step 3 to a medium bowl. Add 1 ounce diced smoked turkey breast and toss to combine. Transfer to a plate. Continue with step 4. Sprinkle with an additional 1/8 teaspoon freshly ground black pepper when serving.

Full recipe: Add 4 ounces diced smoked turkey breast to the salad along with the vinaigrette in step 3 and toss to coat. Continue with step 4. Sprinkle with an additional 1/2 teaspoon freshly ground black pepper when serving.

without
Exchanges/Food Choices: 1/2 Fruit, 1 Vegetable, 1 1/2 Fat
120 calories, 60 calories from fat, 7g total fat, 1g saturated fat, 0g trans fat, 0mg cholesterol, 180mg sodium, 470mg potassium, 16g total carbohydrate, 2g dietary fiber, 10g sugars, 3g protein, 80mg phosphorus

with
Exchanges/Food Choices: 1/2 Fruit, 1 Vegetable, 1 Lean Meat, 1 1/2 Fat
150 calories, 60 calories from fat, 7g total fat, 1g saturated fat, 0g trans fat, 15mg cholesterol, 350mg sodium, 550mg potassium, 16g total carbohydrate, 2g dietary fiber, 10g sugars, 9g protein, 120mg phosphorus

Berry, Basil, and Baby Romaine Salad

Makes 4 servings: 2 cups each

1 1/4 cups fresh or thawed frozen raspberries or wild blueberries, divided

1 large shallot

3 tablespoons unsweetened applesauce

Juice of 1/2 small lemon (1 tablespoon)

1 tablespoon extra-virgin olive oil

1/2 teaspoon freshly ground black pepper, or to taste

1/4 teaspoon + 1/8 teaspoon sea salt, or to taste

5 cups packed baby Romaine lettuce (5 ounces)

1 cup diced unpeeled English cucumber

1/2 cup packed fresh small, whole basil leaves

2 1/2 tablespoons crumbled soft goat cheese

2 tablespoons sliced natural almonds, toasted

When berries are in season in spring and summer, this stunning berry-bursting salad will be sure to strike your fancy. Luckily, you can make it all year long using frozen berries, too. Adorned with fresh basil, dressed in a perky lemon-berry vinaigrette dressing, and accented with natural almonds and more berries, it'll actually seem a bit fancy, too. The bonus: it's more than a bit nutritious.

1. Add 1/2 cup berries, the shallot, applesauce, lemon juice, oil, pepper, and salt to a blender. Cover and purée. Set aside.

2. Arrange the lettuce, cucumber, and basil on 4 individual plates or a large platter. Sprinkle with the berry vinaigrette, the remaining 3/4 cup berries, the goat cheese, and almonds. Adjust seasoning, and serve.

WITH POULTRY, FISH, OR MEAT

One serving: Prepare an outdoor or indoor grill. Brush a 2 1/2-ounce portion of boneless, skinless chicken breast with 1/2 teaspoon extra-virgin olive oil. Grill over direct medium-high heat until well done, about 4 minutes per side. Let stand for 5 minutes. Dice and sprinkle with a pinch of freshly ground black pepper and smidgen of sea salt. Sprinkle the chicken onto one of the salads before topping with the remaining berries, goat cheese, and almonds in step 2.

Full recipe: Prepare an outdoor or indoor grill. Brush two 5-ounce boneless, skinless chicken breasts with 1 teaspoon extra-virgin olive oil each. Grill over direct medium-high heat until well done, about 4–5 minutes per side. Let stand for 5 minutes. Dice and sprinkle with 1/4 teaspoon freshly ground black pepper and 1/8 teaspoon sea salt. Sprinkle the chicken onto the salads before topping with the remaining berries, goat cheese, and almonds in step 2.

without
Exchanges/Food Choices: 1/2 Fruit, 1 Vegetable, 1 Fat
110 calories, 60 calories from fat, 6g total fat, 1.4g saturated fat, 0g trans fat, 0mg cholesterol, 240mg sodium, 270mg potassium, 11g total carbohydrate, 4g dietary fiber, 5g sugars, 3g protein, 70mg phosphorus

with
Exchanges/Food Choices: 1/2 Fruit, 1 Vegetable, 1 1/2 Lean Meat, 1 1/2 Fat
200 calories, 90 calories from fat, 10g total fat, 2g saturated fat, 0g trans fat, 40mg cholesterol, 350mg sodium, 390mg potassium, 11g total carbohydrate, 4g dietary fiber, 5g sugars, 17g protein, 170mg phosphorus

Black Bean and Avocado Cobb Salad

Makes 4 servings: about 2 1/2 cups each

5 cups packed mesclun or mixed baby salad greens (5 ounces)

1 cup grape tomatoes, halved lengthwise

1/2 cup finely diced red onion

1/4 cup sun-dried tomato bits, not oil-packed (rehydrated, if necessary)

1 (15-ounce) can black or kidney beans, gently rinsed and drained (1 1/2 cups)

1 Hass avocado, peeled, pitted, diced

1 ounce enoki, separated, or thinly sliced white button mushrooms

1/4 cup pure-pressed carrot juice

Juice of 1 lime (2 tablespoons) + 1 lime, cut into wedges

1 tablespoon extra-virgin olive oil

1 tablespoon finely chopped fresh tarragon or cilantro, or to taste

1/8 teaspoon + 1/4 teaspoon sea salt, or to taste

1/2 teaspoon freshly ground black pepper, or to taste

There's so much to love about this contemporary Cobb salad. It's a bowl of culinary excitement with an array of veggie textures, colors, and tastes arranged atop a bed of mesclun. Avocado is included for lusciousness. Beans make it hearty. And to top that off, the tarragon-laced carrot vinaigrette is uniquely delicious and makes this Cobb salad no run-of-the-mill recipe.

1. Arrange the mesclun on 4 plates. Top with the grape tomatoes, onion, sun-dried tomato bits, black beans, avocado, and mushrooms.

2. Whisk together the carrot juice, lime juice, oil, tarragon, and 1/8 teaspoon salt in a liquid measuring cup or small bowl.

3. Drizzle the vinaigrette over the salad. Sprinkle with the pepper and remaining 1/4 teaspoon salt, and serve with the lime wedges.

{ WITH POULTRY, FISH, OR MEAT }

One serving: Along with the other toppings, arrange onto one of the salads 2 ounces cubed rotisserie, or roasted, chilled chicken breast meat in step 1. Serve as an entrée salad.

Full recipe: Along with the other toppings, arrange onto the salads 2 ounces each (8 ounces total) cubed rotisserie, or roasted, chilled chicken breast meat in step 1. Serve as an entrée salad.

without
Exchanges/Food Choices: 1 Starch, 1 1/2 Vegetable, 2 Fat
210 calories, 80 calories from fat, 9g total fat, 1.5g saturated fat, 0g trans fat, 0mg cholesterol, 370mg sodium, 820mg potassium, 27g total carbohydrate, 9g dietary fiber, 7g sugars, 8g protein, 170mg phosphorus

with
Exchanges/Food Choices: 1 Starch, 1 1/2 Vegetable, 2 Lean Meat, 2 Fat
300 calories, 100 calories from fat, 11g total fat, 2g saturated fat, 0g trans fat, 50mg cholesterol, 570mg sodium, 1000mg potassium, 28g total carbohydrate, 9g dietary fiber, 7g sugars, 25g protein, 310mg phosphorus

Maitake Powerhouse Salad

Makes 4 servings: 1 1/2 cups salad with
1 large mushroom each

1 1/2 teaspoons grapeseed or
 canola oil

2 (3.5-ounce) fresh maitake
 mushrooms, halved, or 4 portabella
 mushroom caps

1/2 teaspoon freshly ground black
 pepper, divided

1/8 teaspoon sea salt, or to taste

6 cups packed fresh power greens
 (6 ounces)

1 small red onion, halved, very thinly
 sliced

1 1/2 tablespoons white balsamic or
 aged balsamic vinegar

1 tablespoon extra-virgin olive oil

2 tablespoons finely crumbled blue
 cheese or feta cheese

1 1/2 tablespoons raw shelled hemp
 seeds (optional)

Maitake mushrooms, also called hen of the woods, will make this salad an attention grabber. The earthy, tangy, and fresh flavors along with the textures of the salad will keep your attention. The nutritional richness of the greens (try baby spinach, baby kale, and/or chopped chard) will make this recipe one that should be enjoyed often.

1. Heat the grapeseed oil in a large, nonstick skillet over medium-high heat. Add the mushrooms and sauté on all sides until cooked through and browned, about 5–6 minutes. Season with 1/4 teaspoon pepper and the salt.

2. Toss the greens and onion with the vinegar and olive oil in a large bowl. Arrange the salad onto 4 plates. Top with the sautéed mushrooms. Sprinkle with the cheese, hemp seeds (if using), and the remaining 1/4 teaspoon pepper, and serve.

{ WITH POULTRY, FISH, OR MEAT }

One serving: After preparing the mushrooms, add one 2 1/2-ounce portion of lean, grass-fed beef edge of eye steak or filet mignon, about 1 -inch thick, to the nonstick skillet over medium-high heat and pan-cook until medium-rare, about 2 1/2 minutes per side (adjust cooking time based on steak thickness). Let stand at least 5 minutes and season with a pinch each of freshly ground black pepper and sea salt. Thinly slice the steak and arrange onto one of the salads before topping with the maitake.

Full recipe: After preparing the mushrooms, add 4 (2 1/2-ounce) portions of lean, grass-fed beef edge of eye steak or filet mignon, about 1-inch thick each, to the nonstick skillet over medium high heat, and cook until medium-rare, about 2 1/2 minutes per side (adjust cooking time based on steak thickness). Let stand at least 5 minutes. Season with 1/4 teaspoon each freshly ground pepper and sea salt. Thinly slice the steak and arrange on the salads before topping with the maitakes.

without
Exchanges/Food Choices: 1 1/2 Vegetable, 1 1/2 Fat
100 calories, 60 calories from fat, 7g total fat, 1.5g saturated fat, 0g trans fat, 5mg cholesterol, 170mg sodium, 390mg potassium, 8g total carbohydrate, 3g dietary fiber, 3g sugars, 3g protein, 80mg phosphorus

with
Exchanges/Food Choices: 1 1/2 Vegetable, 2 Lean Meat, 2 Fat
190 calories, 90 calories from fat, 10g total fat, 2.5g saturated fat, 0g trans fat, 45mg cholesterol, 330mg sodium, 520mg potassium, 8g total carbohydrate, 3g dietary fiber, 3g sugars, 19g protein, 180mg phosphorus

Niçoise-Style Salad with Edamame

Makes 4 servings: 1/4 recipe each

1 cup frozen shelled edamame

10 ounces baby purple creamer potatoes or fingerling potatoes, unpeeled

1/4 teaspoon sea salt, divided

5 cups packed fresh mixed salad greens (5 ounces)

2 medium yellow vine-ripened tomatoes or Roma tomatoes, cut lengthwise into 12 wedges each

15 pitted Niçoise or kalamata olives, sliced

Juice of 1 lemon (3 tablespoons)

1 1/2 tablespoons extra-virgin olive oil

2 tablespoon chopped fresh tarragon, or to taste

2 tablespoons chopped fresh chives

1/2 teaspoon freshly ground black pepper, or to taste

Salad Niçoise is a traditional French salad in which you'll often find tuna, tomatoes, green beans, and Niçoise olives. I've loosely interpreted the salad here and dressed it in lemony, herbal delight. Edamame provides a protein boost in place of green beans. And tuna is a savory option if you choose. Either way, this sensational salad will satisfy. Every serving will fill up an entire dinner plate!

1. Prepare the edamame according to package directions. Set aside to cool.

2. Place the potatoes in a 9-inch or larger microwave-safe dish, cover with unbleached parchment paper, and microwave on high until tender, about 2 1/2–3 minutes. (Note: Check after 2 minutes and remove any smaller potatoes that are done.) Set aside to cool. Thinly slice and sprinkle with 1/8 teaspoon salt.

3. Arrange the salad greens on individual serving plates. Arrange the potatoes, edamame, tomatoes, and olives on the greens.

4. Whisk together the lemon and oil in a small bowl. Drizzle over the salads. Sprinkle with the tarragon, chives, pepper, and the remaining 1/8 teaspoon salt, and serve.

{ WITH POULTRY, FISH, OR MEAT }

One serving: Prepare an outdoor or indoor grill. Spritz a 2 1/2-ounce portion, about 1 inch thick, of wild yellowfin tuna steak or 1 boneless, skinless chicken thigh with cooking spray. Grill the tuna over high heat until medium-rare or desired doneness, about 1 minute per side, or grill chicken until well done. Add a smidgen of sea salt. Let stand at least 5 minutes. Thinly slice and arrange over one of the salads before drizzling with the lemon vinaigrette in step 4.

Full recipe: Prepare an outdoor or indoor grill. Spritz two 5-ounce wild yellowfin tuna steaks or 4 boneless, skinless chicken thighs with cooking spray. Grill the tuna over high heat until medium-rare or desired doneness, about 1 1/2 minutes per side, or grill chicken until well done. Add 1/8 teaspoon sea salt. Let stand at least 5 minutes. Thinly slice and arrange over the salads before drizzling with the lemon vinaigrette in step 4.

without
Exchanges/Food Choices: 1 1/2 Starch, 1/2 Vegetable, 2 Fat
200 calories, 100 calories from fat, 11g total fat, 1.5g saturated fat, 0g trans fat, 0mg cholesterol, 400mg sodium, 700mg potassium, 20g total carbohydrate, 5g dietary fiber, 3g sugars, 7g protein, 130mg phosphorus

with
Exchanges/Food Choices: 1 Starch, 1/2 Vegetable, 2 Lean Meat, 2 Fat
280 calories, 100 calories from fat, 12g total fat, 1.5g saturated fat, 0g trans fat, 30mg cholesterol, 500mg sodium, 1020mg potassium, 20g total carbohydrate, 5g dietary fiber, 3g sugars, 24g protein, 330mg phosphorus

Summer Squash and Purple Potato Salad

Makes 8 servings: 1 cup each

1 pound baby purple or red creamer potatoes, unpeeled, quartered

1/2 teaspoon sea salt, or to taste

2 medium (8-ounce) yellow summer squash, unpeeled, and quartered lengthwise, cut crosswise into 1/2-inch pieces

6 green asparagus spears, thinly sliced into 1/4-inch "coins"

2/3 cup 4-3-2-1 Dressing (page 83)

1 medium celery stalk, thinly sliced crosswise

1 small jalapeño pepper, with some seeds, minced

3 scallions, green and white parts, thinly sliced on the diagonal

3 tablespoons chopped fresh dill

This isn't any ordinary potato salad. I used summer squash in place of an entire pound of the potatoes to reduce the starchy calories without shrinking serving size or taste. Purple potatoes are the potatoes of choice since they pack a potent nutrient punch—and they are, in fact, purple. Then they're tossed with my versatile and tangy 4-3-2-1 Dressing. It's a surprising addition to your next cookout or picnic.

1. Add the potatoes and salt to a large saucepan and cover with cold water, about 2 inches above the potatoes. Bring to a boil over high heat. Stir in the squash and asparagus, cover, and reduce heat to medium-low. Cook until the potatoes are just tender, about 10 minutes.

2. Drain the vegetable mixture, then immediately, while warm, add to the 4-3-2-1 dressing in a large bowl and stir gently to combine. Chill.

3. Stir in the celery, jalapeño, scallions, and dill. Adjust seasoning, and serve at room temperature or chilled.

One serving: Dice 1/2 ounce lean, uncured Canadian bacon. Heat in a nonstick skillet over medium-high heat until lightly browned, about 1 1/2 minutes. Transfer 1 cup squash-potato salad at serving time to a small serving bowl, sprinkle with the Canadian bacon, and serve.

Full recipe: Dice 4 ounces lean, uncured Canadian bacon. Heat in a nonstick skillet over medium-high heat until lightly browned, about 1 1/2 minutes. At serving time, sprinkle the squash-potato salad with the Canadian bacon, and serve.

without
Exchanges/Food Choices: 1/2 Starch, 1/2 Vegetable, 1 Fat
90 calories, 35 calories from fat, 4g total fat, 0.5g saturated fat, 0g trans fat, 5mg cholesterol, 320mg sodium, 480mg potassium, 13g total carbohydrate, 2g dietary fiber, 3g sugars, 3g protein, 80mg phosphorus

with
Exchanges/Food Choices: 1/2 Starch, 1/2 Vegetable, 1 1/2 Fat
110 calories, 45 calories from fat, 5g total fat, 1g saturated fat, 0g trans fat, 10mg cholesterol, 460mg sodium, 510mg potassium, 13g total carbohydrate, 2g dietary fiber, 3g sugars, 5g protein, 100mg phosphorus

4-3-2-1 Dressing

Makes 8 servings: 1 rounded tablespoon each

Whenever I'm making a potato salad, I use one of the endless versions of my creamy 4-3-2-1 dressing. It works beautifully with the above potato-squash salad or for 2 pounds of potatoes. Below is my favorite well-seasoned version. But you can change the ratios of ingredients, the type of mustard, or swap the lemon juice for various vinegars and use as a creamy dressing for macaroni, tuna, or chicken salad.

1/4 cup plain fat-free Greek yogurt (4 tablespoons)
3 tablespoons mayonnaise
2 tablespoons whole-grain mustard

Juice of 1/2 small lemon (1 tablespoon)
1/2 teaspoon sea salt, or to taste
1/2 teaspoon freshly ground black pepper, or to taste

Whisk together the yogurt, mayonnaise, mustard, lemon juice, salt, and pepper. Makes 2/3 cup. Enjoy in Summer Squash and Purple Potato Salad.

Exchanges/Food Choices: 1 Fat
40 calories, 35 calories from fat, 4g total fat, 0.5g saturated fat, 0g trans fat, 5mg cholesterol, 230mg sodium, 10mg potassium, 1g total carbohydrate, 0g dietary fiber, 0g sugars, 1g protein, 10mg phosphorus

Grilled Bell Pepper, Bok Choy, and Tofu Salad

Makes 4 servings: 1/4 recipe each

1/3 cup brown rice vinegar

1 tablespoon + 1 teaspoon naturally brewed soy sauce

1 tablespoon no-sugar-added apple or apple-peach sauce

1 tablespoon freshly grated gingerroot

2 teaspoons roasted pistachio oil or toasted sesame oil

8 ounces extra-firm tofu, drained and squeezed of excess liquids, cut into 1-inch cubes

2 large red or orange bell peppers, cut into 3/4-inch pieces

3 large (3-ounce) bok choy stalks, halved crosswise

5 cups packed fresh tatsoi or baby lettuce mixture (5 ounces)

3 scallions, green and white parts, minced

2 tablespoons finely chopped roasted unsalted pistachios

3 tablespoons roughly chopped fresh cilantro

Tofu turns into an exciting topping when grilled along with bell peppers and tossed onto this highly flavored Asian salad. The textures, including partly crisp and partly wilted greens, make it extra exciting.

1. Whisk together the vinegar, 1 tablespoon soy sauce, the applesauce, ginger, and oil in a large bowl. Remove 2 tablespoons vinaigrette and reserve. Add the tofu and bell peppers to the vinaigrette in the large bowl. Marinate, gently stirring occasionally, for 30 minutes.

2. Prepare an outdoor or indoor grill. Insert the tofu and bell peppers onto separate reusable or water-soaked bamboo skewers, allowing some space between each tofu cube and bell pepper piece for best grilled results. Dip the bok choy (both the top leaf portions and bottom stalk portions) into the remaining marinade in the large bowl to lightly coat.

3. Grill (in batches, if necessary) the tofu skewers, bell pepper skewers, and the bok choy over medium-high heat until lightly charred and the peppers are just tender, turning only as needed, about 1 minute for the leafy portion of bok choy and 8 minutes for the skewers and bottom portion of bok choy. Remove from the grill. Thinly slice the bok choy, and remove the tofu and peppers from the skewers.

4. Arrange the tatsoi, bok choy, and scallions onto 4 plates. Top with the bell peppers and tofu. Drizzle with the reserved 2 tablespoons vinaigrette and the remaining 1 teaspoon soy sauce. Sprinkle with the pistachios and cilantro, and serve at room temperature.

WITH POULTRY, FISH, OR MEAT

One serving: In place of 2 ounces tofu, cut 1 1/2 ounces pork tenderloin into 6 cubes. Toss in any remaining marinade after coating the bok choy in step 2. Insert onto a skewer and grill next to or after the vegetables until medium or medium-well done, about 2 minutes. Arrange the grilled pork cubes onto one of the salads in place of the tofu in step 4.

Full recipe: In place of the tofu, cut 6 ounces pork tenderloin into 24 cubes. Toss in the marinade in place of the tofu in step 1. Insert onto skewers and grill next to the vegetables until medium or medium-well done, about 2 minutes. Arrange the grilled pork cubes onto the salads in place of the tofu in step 4.

without
Exchanges/Food Choices: 2 Vegetable, 1 Medium-Fat Meat, 1/2 Fat
180 calories, 70 calories from fat, 8g total fat, 1g saturated fat, 0g trans fat, 0mg cholesterol, 460mg sodium, 990mg potassium, 17g total carbohydrate, 5g dietary fiber, 10g sugars, 12g protein, 220mg phosphorus

with
Exchanges/Food Choices: 2 Vegetable, 1 Lean Meat, 1 Fat
170 calories, 50 calories from fat, 6g total fat, 1g saturated fat, 0g trans fat, 20mg cholesterol, 480mg sodium, 1040mg potassium, 16g total carbohydrate, 5g dietary fiber, 10g sugars, 15g protein, 220mg phosphorus

Keep Your Cool

For many centuries, herbs and spices have been used for medicinal purposes, notably in Asia, India, and Mexico. Fresh cilantro and gingerroot, for instance, were consumed to keep internal body heat balanced during the excessive heat of the summer months. So recipes like this one will excite your taste buds all year round, but may also help keep you comfortable in warm weather.

Couscous Salad with Arugula, Feta, and Roasted Fig

Makes 6 servings: 1 cup each

1 cup dry whole-wheat couscous

Juice of 1 lemon (3 tablespoons), divided

2 tablespoons extra-virgin olive oil, divided

3/4 teaspoon sea salt, or to taste

3/4 teaspoon freshly ground black pepper, or to taste

6 fresh Black Mission or Brown Turkey figs

Cooking spray

2 1/2 cups packed fresh baby arugula (2.5 ounces)

1/4 cup toasted pine nuts

2 tablespoons finely crumbled feta cheese, divided

3 tablespoons thinly sliced fresh basil + 6 small basil sprigs for garnish

1 teaspoon finely chopped fresh rosemary, or to taste

Couscous is one of the quickest grain foods to fix. But that doesn't mean it needs to be served just as a quick side. Here's a salad that gives it glitz. It's basically a culinary coupling of a simple grain side and a spectacular leafy salad, but the highlight is the roasted figs. Select this recipe when fresh figs are seasonal in summer or early fall. Or prepare this salad in winter or springtime with two roasted pears cut into wedges. It's lovely and a bit luxurious!

1. Cook the couscous according to package directions. Immediately stir in 2 tablespoons lemon juice and fluff with a fork. Transfer the couscous to a large bowl, sprinkle with 1 tablespoon oil, the salt, and pepper, and stir to combine. Set aside to cool for 30 minutes, stirring occasionally to prevent sticking. Then chill in the refrigerator.

2. Meanwhile, preheat the oven to 375°F. Spritz the fresh figs with cooking spray and arrange on a small baking pan. Roast until the figs are glossy and softened, about 12 minutes. Let stand for about 30 minutes to cool. Then chill in the refrigerator. Gently slice each fig into quarters lengthwise and remove stems.

3. Stir the arugula, pine nuts, 1 tablespoon feta cheese, the sliced basil, rosemary, and the remaining 1 tablespoon lemon juice and 1 tablespoon oil into the cool couscous. Gently stir in about three-fourths of the quartered figs. Adjust seasoning.

4. Transfer the couscous salad to individual salad plates or bowls. Arrange the remaining figs on top and sprinkle with the remaining 1 tablespoon feta. Garnish with the basil sprigs, and serve at room temperature.

{ WITH POULTRY, FISH, OR MEAT }

One serving: Sprinkle 2/3 ounce precooked, chilled, diced poultry sausage link onto one of the couscous servings in step 4.

Full recipe: Stir 4 ounces precooked, chilled, diced poultry sausage links into the couscous in step 3.

without
Exchanges/Food Choices: 2 Starch, 1/2 Fruit, 2 Fat
240 calories, 90 calories from fat, 10g total fat,
1.5g saturated fat, 0g trans fat, 5mg cholesterol,
330mg sodium, 260mg potassium, 36g total
carbohydrate, 6g dietary fiber, 10g sugars,
7g protein, 110mg phosphorus

with
Exchanges/Food Choices: 2 Starch, 1/2 Fruit,
1/2 Medium-Fat Meat, 2 Fat
270 calories, 100 calories from fat, 12g total fat,
2g saturated fat, 0g trans fat, 15mg cholesterol,
560mg sodium, 300mg potassium, 37g total
carbohydrate, 6g dietary fiber, 10g sugars,
10g protein, 140mg phosphorus

1/3 cup plain fat-free Greek yogurt

1/4 cup Major Grey's mango chutney

1 1/2 tablespoons hot Madras curry powder, or to taste

1 tablespoon mayonnaise or vegan mayonnaise

1 1/2 teaspoons freshly grated gingerroot, or to taste

1 teaspoon apple cider vinegar

1/4 teaspoon + 1/8 teaspoon sea salt

1/2 cup finely diced fennel bulb

1 scallion, green and white parts, minced

2 tablespoons chopped fresh cilantro

1 (14-ounce) package extra-firm tofu, drained and squeezed of excess liquid, diced

without
Exchanges/Food Choices: 1/2 Carbohydrate, 1 Medium-Fat Meat, 1 Fat
160 calories, 80 calories from fat, 9g total fat, 1g saturated fat, 0g trans fat, 0mg cholesterol, 270mg sodium, 250mg potassium, 11g total carbohydrate, 2g dietary fiber, 6g sugars, 12g protein, 180mg phosphorus

with
Exchanges/Food Choices: 1/2 Carbohydrate, 2 Lean Meat, 1/2 Fat
170 calories, 50 calories from fat, 5g total fat, 1g saturated fat, 0g trans fat, 60mg cholesterol, 480mg sodium, 310mg potassium, 9g total carbohydrate, 2g dietary fiber, 6g sugars, 21g protein, 200mg phosphorus

Hot Madras Curried Tofu Salad

Makes 4 servings: 2/3 cup each

If you're into flavor, you'll be into this simple-to-fix salad. Enjoy the curried tofu recipe just like chicken salad. Try it on thick slices of beefsteak or heirloom tomato or serve with whole-grain brown rice crackers, if you like.

1. Stir together the yogurt, chutney, curry powder, mayonnaise, ginger, vinegar, and salt in a medium bowl until well combined. Stir in the fennel, scallion, and cilantro until combined. Stir in the tofu until well combined.

2. Adjust seasoning, and serve.

WITH POULTRY, FISH, OR MEAT

One serving: Before adding the tofu, transfer 1/4 cup curry mixture to a small bowl. Dice 2 1/4 ounces rotisserie, or roasted, chilled chicken breast and stir into the mixture in the small bowl. Stir 10 1/2 ounces instead of 14 ounces diced tofu into the curry mixture in the medium bowl.

Full recipe: Dice 9 ounces rotisserie, or roasted, chilled chicken breast. Stir into the salad instead of the 14 ounces tofu.

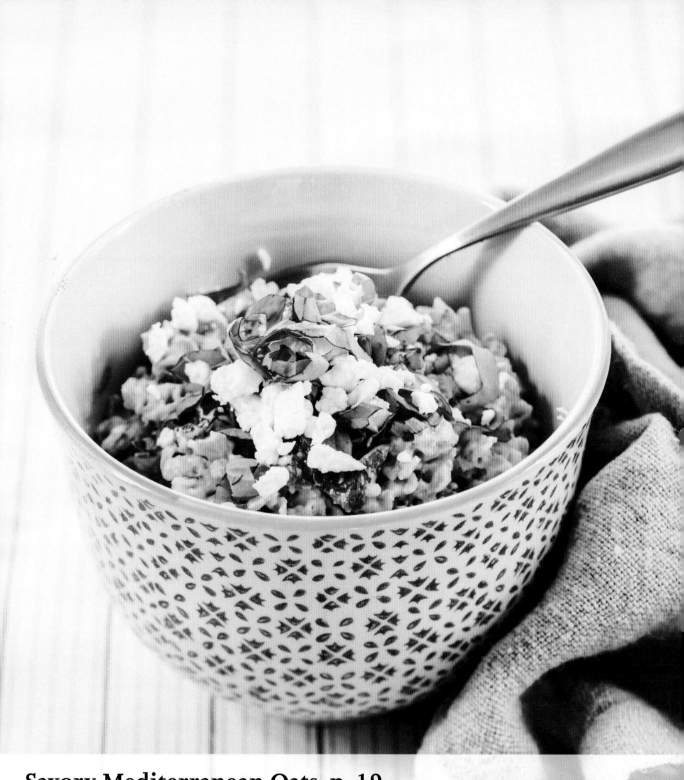

Savory Mediterranean Oats, p. 19

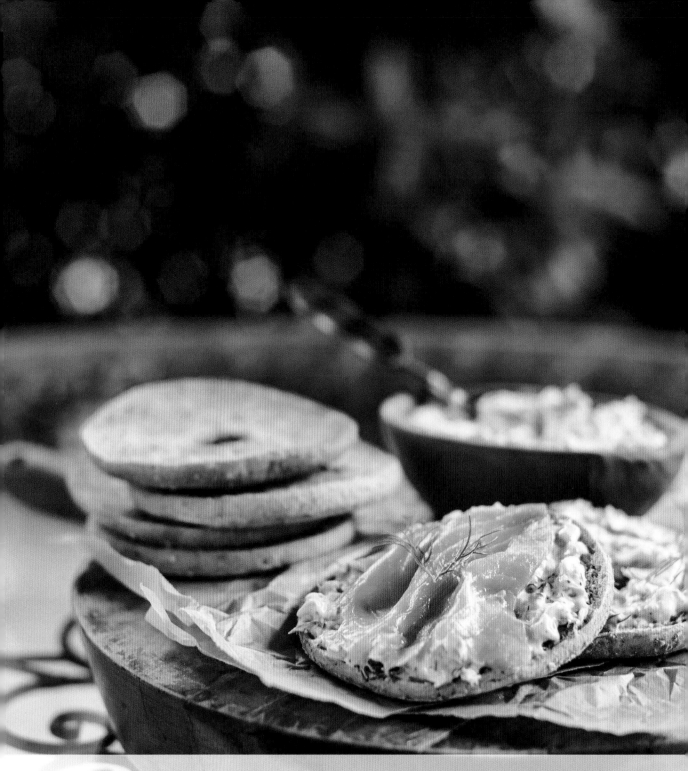

Open–Face Bagel Thins with Scallion Schmear, p. 30

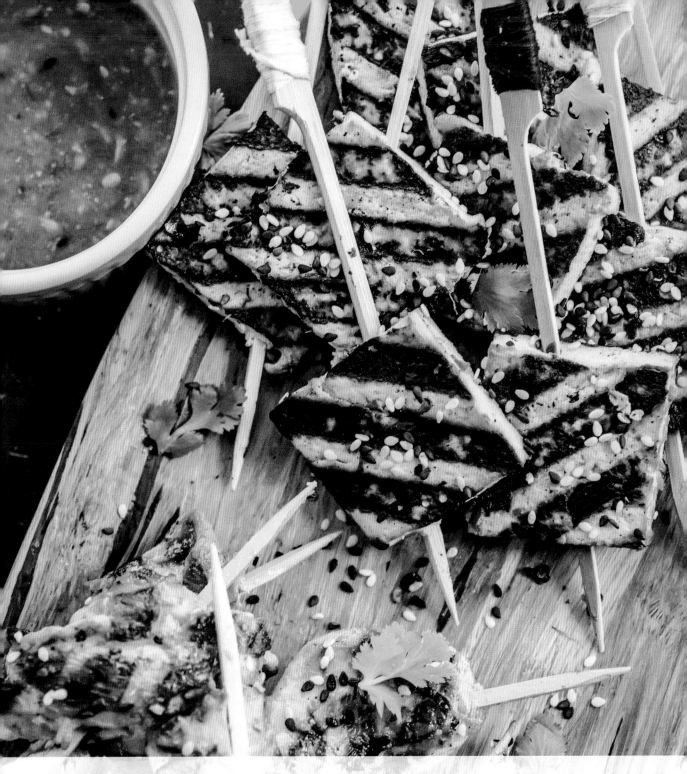

Pan-Grilled Tofu Skewers, p. 42

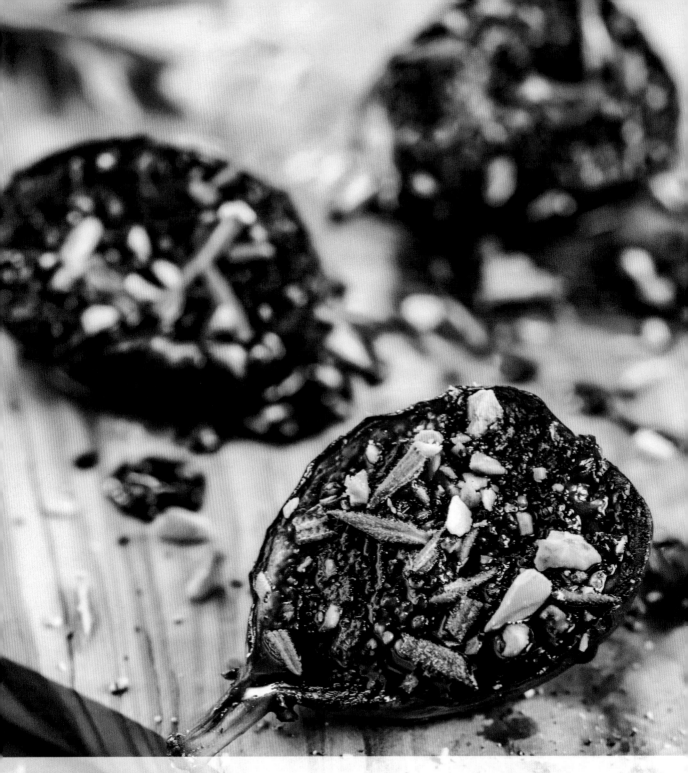

Grilled Figs with Balsamic Reduction, p. 52

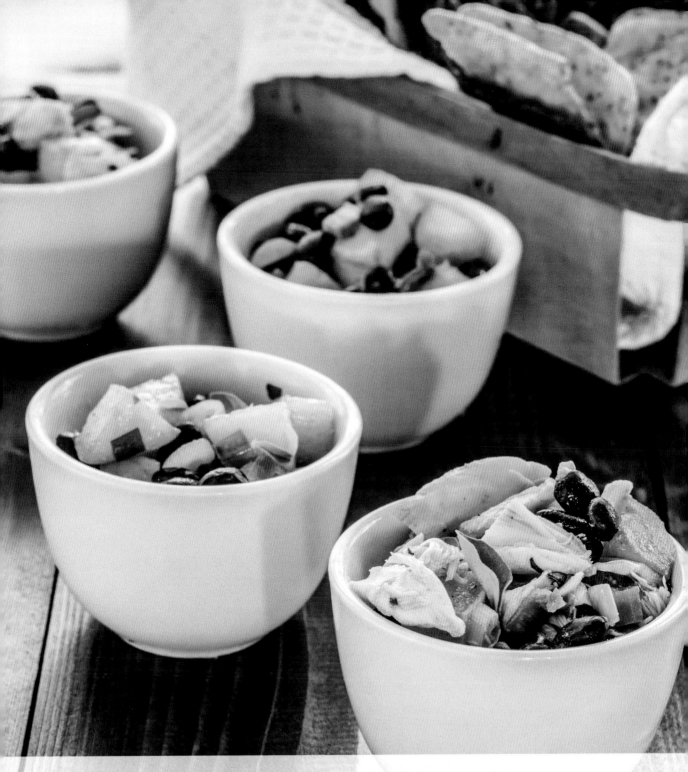

Peach and Black Bean Salsa with Chips, p. 64

Peppercorn Pistachio Caesar-Style Salad, p. 68

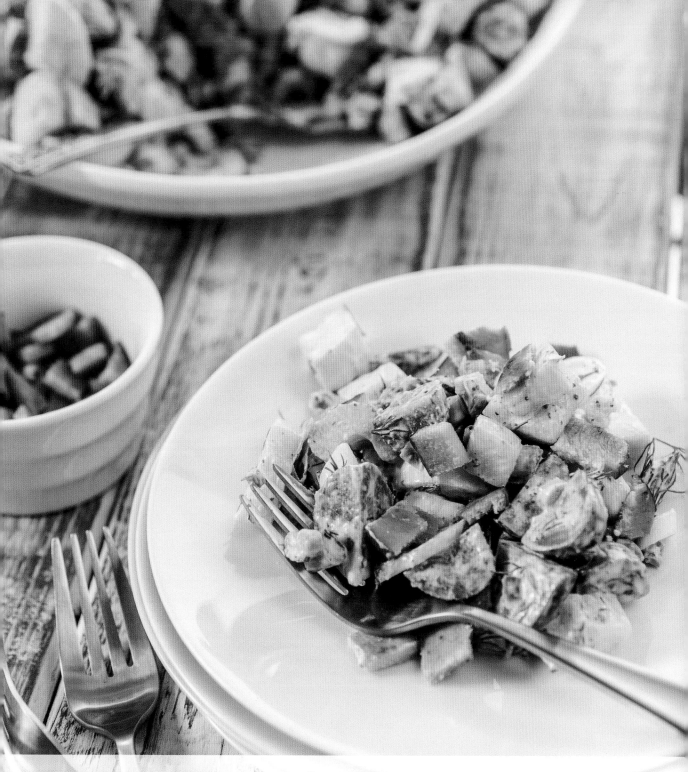

Summer Squash and Purple Potato Salad, p. 82

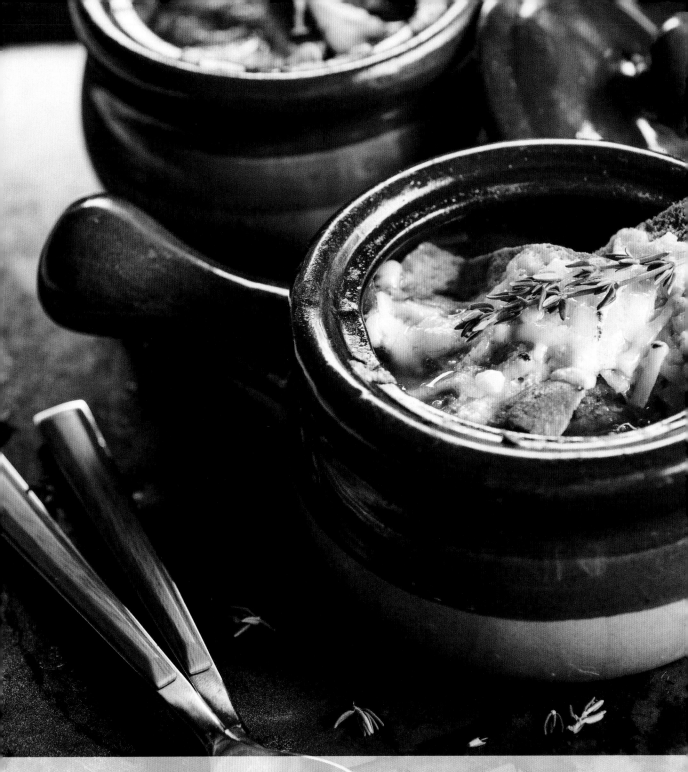

Red Onion Soup with Shiitake Broth, p. 106

Orzo Trail Mix Salad

Makes 6 servings: 1 cup each

Here's a leafy orzo salad that's a culinary hit! There's something in it for everyone. The trail mix addition makes it playful. So play around with different trail mix combinations of dried fruits, nuts, and seeds to find your favorite. My choice: black seedless raisins, roasted pistachios, and sunflower seeds.

1. Cook the orzo according to package directions. Drain.

2. Meanwhile, whisk together the lemon juice, oil, salt, and pepper in a large bowl until combined. Add the hot orzo to the lemon vinaigrette and stir to coat. Set aside to cool for about 30 minutes, stirring occasionally to prevent sticking. Then chill in the refrigerator.

3. Gently stir the mizuna, trail mix, artichoke hearts, basil, and desired amount of the lemon zest into the cool orzo until the mizuna is moistened. Adjust seasoning.

4. Arrange the orzo salad in bowls, and serve at room temperature.

{ WITH POULTRY, FISH, OR MEAT }

One serving: Finely dice a 1-ounce grilled, organic chicken thigh strip and stir into one of the servings of orzo salad in step 4. Alternatively, break apart 1 ounce canned, drained, oil-packed wild Pacific sardines into bite-size pieces and stir into the serving.

Full recipe: Finely dice 6 ounces grilled, organic chicken thighs and stir into each of the servings of orzo salad in step 4. Alternatively, break apart 6 ounces canned, drained, oil-packed wild Pacific sardines into bite-size pieces and stir into the salad.

1 cup dry whole-wheat orzo

Juice and zest of 1 lemon (3 tablespoons juice)

1 tablespoon flaxseed or extra-virgin olive oil

3/4 teaspoon sea salt, or to taste

3/4 teaspoon freshly ground black pepper, or to taste

4 cups packed fresh mizuna or baby lettuce mixture (4 ounces)

3/4 cup unsalted trail mix or mixture of dried fruit and nuts and/or seeds

1/2 cup finely diced, drained, marinated artichoke hearts

1/4 cup thinly sliced fresh basil

without
Exchanges/Food Choices: 2 Starch, 1 Vegetable, 1 1/2 Fat
250 calories, 80 calories from fat, 9g total fat, 1.5g saturated fat, 0g trans fat, 0mg cholesterol, 340mg sodium, 260mg potassium, 38g total carbohydrate, 4g dietary fiber, 1g sugars, 9g protein, 170mg phosphorus

with
Exchanges/Food Choices: 2 Starch, 1 Vegetable, 1 Lean Meat, 2 Fat
310 calories, 110 calories from fat, 12g total fat, 2g saturated fat, 0g trans fat, 40mg cholesterol, 480mg sodium, 370mg potassium, 38g total carbohydrate, 4g dietary fiber, 1g sugars, 16g protein, 310mg phosphorus

Creamy Picnic at the Pops Pasta Salad

Makes 8 servings: 3/4 cup each

8 ounces dry whole-wheat or other whole-grain penne pasta

3 tablespoons mayonnaise

2 tablespoons plain fat-free Greek yogurt

2 teaspoons apple cider vinegar

1 1/2 teaspoons whole-grain Dijon mustard

1/2 teaspoon finely chopped fresh rosemary, or to taste

1/4 teaspoon ground cayenne pepper, or to taste

1/2 cup fresh or thawed frozen peas

1/3 cup sun-dried tomatoes, not oil-packed, thinly sliced (rehydrated, if necessary)

10 cornichons (midget gherkins), very thinly sliced into "coins"

1 medium freshly roasted yellow or orange bell pepper, finely diced (page 91)

1/4 cup finely diced red onion

1/4 teaspoon + 1/8 teaspoon sea salt, or to taste

Move over, old-fashioned macaroni salad. Here's a kicked up, party-friendlier, creamy pasta salad ready for the making. The pops of sweet peas, fragrant rosemary, and perky sun-dried tomatoes make it extra special and extra nutritious. Serve it up at a large picnic gathering or causal backyard cookout.

1. Cook the pasta according to package directions. Drain the pasta, toss or stir the pasta in the saucepan with several ice cubes to cool, or rinse under cold running water, and drain again.

2. Meanwhile, whisk together the mayonnaise, yogurt, vinegar, mustard, rosemary, and cayenne in a large serving bowl.

3. Add the pasta, peas, sun-dried tomatoes, cornichons, bell pepper, and onion, and stir until well combined. Add the salt, adjust seasoning, and serve.

{ WITH POULTRY, FISH, OR MEAT }

One serving: Transfer 3/4 cup pasta salad in step 3 to a small bowl or salad plate before serving. Sprinkle on or stir 1 ounce diced, lean, uncured ham into this individual serving.

Full recipe: Stir 8 ounces diced, lean, uncured ham into the recipe in step 3.

without
Exchanges/Food Choices: 1 1/2 Starch, 1/2 Vegetable, 1 Fat
170 calories, 40 calories from fat, 4.5g total fat, 0.5g saturated fat, 0g trans fat, 0mg cholesterol, 230mg sodium, 190mg potassium, 30g total carbohydrate, 4g dietary fiber, 5g sugars, 6g protein, 100mg phosphorus

with
Exchanges/Food Choices: 1 1/2 Starch, 1/2 Vegetable, 1 Lean Meat, 1 Fat
200 calories, 45 calories from fat, 5g total fat, 1g saturated fat, 0g trans fat, 20mg cholesterol, 390mg sodium, 280mg potassium, 30g total carbohydrate, 4g dietary fiber, 6g sugars, 12g protein, 160mg phosphorus

Freshly Roasted Peppers

Stand up each bell pepper and cut down each side, creating 4 large, wide pieces. Slice off the bottom of the pepper, creating another piece. Discard the stem and seeds. Line a baking sheet with recycled aluminum foil and arrange the pepper slices in a single layer, skin side up. Broil about 3 inches from the heat source, until the skins are well charred. Alternatively, carefully char the whole pepper over an open flame, such as a gas burner flame. Transfer the well-charred pepper to a bowl, cover, and let stand to complete the cooking process, about 10 minutes. Rub off all or most of the charred skin.

Italian Rotini and Grilled Vegetable Salad

Makes 6 servings: 1 1/3 cups each

1 medium (1-pound) eggplant, unpeeled, cut into 1/2-inch rounds

1 medium (7-ounce) zucchini, unpeeled, and cut into 4 lengthwise slices

1 medium red onion, peeled, trimmed, and cut crosswise into 4 thick rounds (do not separate into rings)

1 small fennel bulb with core, stems and fronds removed, cut into 4 slices

3 tablespoons extra-virgin olive oil, divided

5 ounces whole-wheat or other whole-grain rotini pasta

3 tablespoons red wine vinegar

2 large garlic cloves, minced or creamed

1/8 teaspoon + 3/4 teaspoon sea salt

1/2 teaspoon freshly ground black pepper, or to taste

1/3 cup thinly sliced fresh basil

Being an Italian pasta salad fan for nearly my entire life, I'm always creating new versions to stay fresh. Here's one that excites the taste buds. It's laden with grilled vegetables such as eggplant, zucchini, onion, and fennel, which makes it super tasty and satisfying and also keeps total carbs in check. The generous finish of fresh basil provides fragrant delight in every bite.

1. Prepare an outdoor or indoor grill. Lightly brush the eggplant, zucchini, onion, and fennel slices with 1 tablespoon of the oil. Grill over direct medium-high heat until fully cooked and rich grill marks form, about 5 minutes per side, turning only as needed. Set aside.

2. Cook the pasta according to package directions. Drain the pasta, toss or stir the pasta in the saucepan with several ice cubes to cool, or rinse under cold running water, and drain again.

3. Meanwhile, whisk together the vinegar, the remaining 2 tablespoons oil, the garlic, 1/8 teaspoon salt, and the pepper in a large serving bowl. Add the drained pasta, and toss to coat.

4. Dice the eggplant, zucchini, and onion; finely dice the fennel. Season with the remaining 3/4 teaspoon salt. Stir the vegetables and basil into the pasta until just combined. Adjust seasoning, and serve.

{ WITH POULTRY, FISH, OR MEAT }

One serving: Brush a 2-ounce portion of skin-on wild Alaskan sockeye salmon or farmed Arctic char fillets with 1/2 teaspoon extra-virgin olive oil. Grill next to the vegetables, or after the vegetables, until cooked through, about 4 minutes per side, turning only once. Peel off the skin and flake into small bite-size pieces. Sprinkle with a smidgen of sea salt. Toss into the pasta salad in step 4 before adjusting seasoning.

Full recipe: Brush two 6-ounce skin-on wild Alaskan salmon or farmed Arctic char fillets with 1 tablespoon extra-virgin olive oil. Grill next to the vegetables, or after the vegetables, until cooked through, about 4 1/2 minutes per side, turning only once. Peel off the skin and flake into small, bite-size pieces. Sprinkle with 1/8 teaspoon sea salt. Toss into the pasta salad in step 4 before adjusting seasoning.

without
Exchanges/Food Choices: 1 1/2 Starch,
1 Vegetable, 1 Fat
180 calories, 70 calories from fat, 8g total fat,
1g saturated fat, 0g trans fat, 0mg cholesterol,
360mg sodium, 450mg potassium, 27g total
carbohydrate, 5g dietary fiber, 4g sugars,
5g protein, 110mg phosphorus

with
Exchanges/Food Choices: 1 1/2 Starch,
1 Vegetable, 1 Lean Meat, 2 Fat
280 calories, 110 calories from fat, 12g total fat,
2g saturated fat, 0g trans fat, 25mg cholesterol,
440mg sodium, 700mg potassium, 28g total
carbohydrate, 6g dietary fiber, 5g sugars,
17g protein, 270mg phosphorus

Scrubbed Produce

I recommend leaving the edible peel/skin on most veggies and fruits. That's because it can provide a boost of texture, color, and overall nutrition, including fiber, to a recipe. Whenever you plan to use unpeeled conventional produce in a recipe, be sure to clean and scrub it well before preparation to reduce or remove harmful pesticide residue, dirt, and grit. Scrub organic produce well, too.

Lemon-Herb Farro and Spinach Salad

Makes 4 servings: 1 rounded cup each

Farro is a nutty, chewy whole grain that provides heartiness and staying power to this minty salad with Grecian flair. The spinach provides freshness and makes the portion size bigger. Your palate will be pleasantly pleased, too.

2/3 cup whole farro, rinsed and drained

1/2 teaspoon sea salt, divided

2 tablespoons plain fat-free Greek yogurt

Juice of 1/2 lemon (1 1/2 tablespoons)

2 tablespoons extra-virgin olive oil

2 tablespoons finely chopped fresh mint

1 large garlic clove, minced

3/4 teaspoon freshly ground black pepper, or to taste

1 cup grape tomatoes, halved lengthwise

2 scallions, green and white parts, thinly sliced

3/4 cup extra-thin slices unpeeled English cucumber ("coins")

3 cups packed fresh baby spinach or mesclun (3 ounces)

1. Combine 3 cups water and the farro in a small saucepan, and bring to a boil over high heat. Reduce the heat to low, cover, and simmer until the farro is desired tenderness, about 40 minutes. Drain well.

2. Transfer the farro to a medium bowl. Stir in 1/4 teaspoon salt and set aside to cool for about 30 minutes, stirring occasionally to prevent sticking. Then chill in the refrigerator.

3. Whisk together the yogurt, lemon juice, oil, mint, garlic, pepper, and the remaining 1/4 teaspoon salt until combined in a large bowl. Add the cool farro and stir to combine. Add the tomatoes, scallions, and cucumber, and toss to combine. Add the spinach and toss well to combine. Adjust seasoning, and serve on individual plates or in bowls.

{ WITH POULTRY, FISH, OR MEAT }

One serving: Top one of the servings with three 1/2-ounce strips of grilled chicken breast or 3 large cooked shrimp. Sprinkle generously with freshly ground black pepper to taste.

Full recipe: Stir 6 ounces grilled chicken breast cubes into the farro salad in step 3. Or top each serving with three 1/2-ounce strips of grilled chicken breast or 3 large cooked shrimp. Sprinkle generously with freshly ground black pepper to taste.

without
Exchanges/Food Choices: 1 1/2 Starch, 1 Vegetable, 1 1/2 Fat
190 calories, 70 calories from fat, 8g total fat, 1g saturated fat, 0g trans fat, 0mg cholesterol, 310mg sodium, 370mg potassium, 27g total carbohydrate, 4g dietary fiber, 3g sugars, 6g protein, 140mg phosphorus

with
Exchanges/Food Choices: 1 1/2 Starch, 1 Vegetable, 2 Lean Meat, 1/2 Fat
260 calories, 80 calories from fat, 10g total fat, 1.5g saturated fat, 0g trans fat, 35mg cholesterol, 350mg sodium, 480mg potassium, 27g total carbohydrate, 4g dietary fiber, 3g sugars, 19g protein, 240mg phosphorus

Orange and Herb Quinoa Salad

Makes 4 servings: 3/4 cup each

1 cup low-sodium vegetable broth

1/2 cup freshly squeezed orange juice + 2 teaspoons orange zest

3/4 cup quinoa, rinsed and drained

Juice of 1/2 lemon (1 1/2 tablespoons)

2 teaspoons grapeseed or extra-virgin olive oil

1/4 teaspoon + 1/8 teaspoon sea salt, or to taste

1/4 cup chopped fresh mint

1/4 cup chopped fresh basil

3 tablespoons sliced natural almonds, toasted

without
Exchanges/Food Choice: 1 1/2 Starch, 1 Fat
180 calories, 60 calories from fat,
6g total fat, 0.5g saturated fat, 0g trans fat,
0mg cholesterol, 260mg sodium,
300mg potassium, 26g total carbohydrate,
3g dietary fiber, 5g sugars, 6g protein,
180mg phosphorus

with
Exchanges/Food Choices: 1 1/2 Starch,
2 Lean Meat
210 calories, 60 calories from fat,
7g total fat, 0.5g saturated fat, 0g trans fat,
15mg cholesterol, 430mg sodium,
380mg potassium, 26g total carbohydrate,
3g dietary fiber, 5g sugars, 12g protein,
220mg phosphorus

When citrus is added to quinoa, get ready to be enticed. When generously accessorized with a fresh herb "potpourri" and toasty almonds, a beautiful and satisfying salad is the result. Grow fresh mint and basil indoors to enjoy this refreshing salad all year long.

1. Bring the broth and orange juice to a boil in a small saucepan over high heat. Stir in the quinoa. Cover, reduce heat to low, and cook until the quinoa is nearly tender, about 20 minutes. Remove from heat and let stand, covered, for 5 minutes to complete the cooking process. Transfer to a large bowl. Set aside to cool for about 30 minutes, stirring occasionally to prevent sticking. Then chill in the refrigerator.

2. Meanwhile, whisk together the lemon juice, oil, and salt in a small bowl. Stir the lemon vinaigrette into the chilled quinoa until well combined. Stir in the mint and basil. Adjust seasoning.

3. Transfer the quinoa salad to individual bowls, sprinkle with the almonds and orange zest, and serve.

WITH POULTRY, FISH, OR MEAT

One serving: After adjusting seasoning in step 2, transfer 3/4 cup quinoa mixture to a small bowl. Dice 1 ounce herb-roasted turkey breast and stir into the quinoa mixture.

Full recipe: After adjusting seasoning in step 2, dice 4 ounces herb-roasted turkey breast and stir into the quinoa mixture.

Tarragon White Bean Salad

Makes 3 servings: 1/2 cup each

Canned cannellini beans are a key pantry staple. Their protein and fiber make them especially satiating. They're versatile in cuisine, too. Cannellini beans can be whirled into recipes to provide creaminess without cream, and they can be sensational in a starring role like in this bean salad. The addition of fresh tarragon makes this simply prepared recipe special.

1. Whisk together the vinegar, oil, mustard, tarragon, and pepper in a medium bowl. Add the beans and shallot, and toss to combine.

2. Serve in individual bowls. Garnish, if desired, with additional fresh tarragon leaves.

{ WITH POULTRY, FISH, OR MEAT }

One serving: Finely chop 1/3 slice of cooked, hardwood-smoked, uncured turkey bacon or Sunday bacon and toss onto one of the servings.

Full recipe: Finely chop 1 slice of cooked, hardwood-smoked, uncured turkey bacon or Sunday bacon and toss into the salad before transferring to individual bowls.

1 1/2 tablespoons white balsamic or white wine vinegar

1 1/2 tablespoons extra-virgin olive oil

1 teaspoon Dijon mustard

1 teaspoon chopped fresh tarragon

1/8 teaspoon freshly ground black pepper, or to taste

1 (15-ounce) can cannellini or other white beans, gently rinsed and drained (1 1/2 cups)

1 small shallot, minced

without
Exchanges/Food Choices: 1 1/2 Starch, 2 Lean Meat
190 calories, 60 calories from fat, 7g total fat, 1g saturated fat, 0g trans fat, 0mg cholesterol, 400mg sodium, 500mg potassium, 24g total carbohydrate, 7g dietary fiber, 4g sugars, 9g protein, 100mg phosphorus

with
Exchanges/Food Choices: 1 1/2 Starch, 2 Lean Meat
200 calories, 60 calories from fat, 8g total fat, 1g saturated fat, 0g trans fat, 10mg cholesterol, 460mg sodium, 510mg potassium, 24g total carbohydrate, 7g dietary fiber, 4g sugars, 11g protein, 110mg phosphorus

Barley Tabbouli Salad with Caramelized Shallot

Makes 4 servings: 3/4 rounded cup each

1/2 cup whole hull-less barley (not pearled barley), rinsed

Juice of 1/2 lemon (1 1/2 tablespoons)

2 tablespoons extra-virgin olive oil, divided

1/2 teaspoon sea salt, divided

1/2 teaspoon freshly ground black pepper, divided

3 large shallots, finely diced

2 large garlic cloves, minced

3/4 cup Persian or English cucumber, unpeeled, finely diced

1 medium vine-ripened tomato, pulp removed, finely diced

2 scallions, green and white parts, thinly sliced

1/3 cup finely chopped fresh flat-leaf parsley

3 tablespoons finely chopped fresh mint

Tabbouli is the salad that I grew up on. I adore it when traditionally prepared, but I get a kick out of changing the recipe up for extra temptation. So here's one of those creations: using barley instead of bulgur and incorporating caramelized shallot to add flavor depth. You'll love the nuttier texture it gives this nontraditional tabbouli.

1. Bring the barley and 2 1/4 cups water to a boil in a medium saucepan over high heat. Reduce heat to low, cover, and simmer until the barley is chewy yet tender, about 45 minutes. Remove from heat and let stand for 10 minutes, covered, to complete the cooking process. Drain well of any excess liquid.

2. Whisk together the lemon juice, 1 tablespoon oil, and 1/4 teaspoon each salt and pepper in a medium bowl until combined. Add the hot, drained barley and stir to coat. Set aside to cool for about 30 minutes, stirring occasionally to prevent sticking. Then chill in the refrigerator.

3. Meanwhile, heat 1/2 tablespoon oil in a large, nonstick skillet over medium-high heat. Add the shallots and sauté until well caramelized, about 5 minutes. Stir in the garlic and sauté for 30 seconds. Transfer to a small bowl

4. Stir the cucumber, tomato, scallions, parsley, mint, and the remaining 1/2 tablespoon oil and 1/4 teaspoon salt and pepper into the cool barley. Stir in the shallot mixture. Adjust seasoning, and serve in individual bowls.

WITH POULTRY, FISH, OR MEAT

One serving: Stir 1 1/4 ounces flaked, canned, water-packed white, low-mercury Albacore tuna into one of the servings in step 4.

Full recipe: Stir 5 ounces flaked, canned, water-packed, white, low-mercury Albacore tuna into the cool barley at the beginning of step 4.

without
Exchanges/Food Choices: 1 1/2 Starch, 1 Vegetable, 1 Fat
180 calories, 70 calories from fat, 8g total fat, 1g saturated fat, 0g trans fat, 0mg cholesterol, 300mg sodium, 390mg potassium, 27g total carbohydrate, 6g dietary fiber, 4g sugars, 5g protein, 100mg phosphorus

with
Exchanges/Food Choices: 1 Starch, 2 Vegetable, 1 Lean Meat, 1 Fat
220 calories, 70 calories from fat, 8g total fat, 1g saturated fat, 0g trans fat, 15mg cholesterol, 390mg sodium, 450mg potassium, 27g total carbohydrate, 6g dietary fiber, 4g sugars, 12g protein, 150mg phosphorus

Roasted Carrot, Cippolini, and Dill Rice Salad

Makes 4 servings: 2/3 cup each

2/3 cup short-grain brown rice

1 tablespoon + 1 teaspoon extra-virgin olive oil

2 medium carrots, very thinly sliced crosswise (about 1/8-inch thick)

3 peeled cippolini onions, cut into 8 wedges each (2 ounces)

Juice of 1/2 lemon (1 1/2 tablespoons)

1/2 teaspoon sea salt, or to taste

1/2 teaspoon freshly ground black pepper, or to taste

1 tablespoon chopped fresh dill

When making pilaf, long-grain rice is my pick. When making a rice salad, the nubbier short-grain rice stands up nicely. Combine it with the classic pairing of carrots and dill, and you'll find this salad to be exceptional. Keep this recipe on-the-ready for incorporating leftover holiday turkey or chicken.

1. Preheat the oven to 425°F. Cook the rice according to package directions. Transfer to a large bowl. Stir in 1 teaspoon oil and set aside to cool for about 30 minutes, stirring occasionally to help prevent sticking. Chill in the refrigerator.

2. Meanwhile, add the carrots and onions to a medium bowl. Drizzle with 1/2 tablespoon oil and toss to coat. Transfer to a large, nonstick baking sheet, arrange in a single layer, and roast until the vegetables are tender and lightly caramelized, about 17 minutes.

3. Whisk together the lemon juice, the remaining 1/2 tablespoon oil, the salt, and pepper in a small bowl. Stir the vinaigrette and chopped dill into the rice. Then stir in the carrots and onions. Adjust seasoning.

4. Serve on individual plates or in bowls. If desired, garnish with lemon wedges from the remaining 1/2 lemon.

{ WITH POULTRY, FISH, OR MEAT }

One serving: Stir 2 1/2 ounces chopped, roasted, chilled turkey or chicken breast plus 1/4 teaspoon freshly ground black pepper into one serving along with the carrots, onion, and dill in step 3. (Hint: Use holiday turkey or chicken leftovers.) Alternatively, place about a 2 1/2-ounce piece of wild Pacific halibut fillet onto an 8-inch square baking pan lined with unbleached parchment paper. Brush with 3/4 teaspoon extra-virgin olive oil and season with a smidgen of sea salt and freshly ground black pepper, or to taste. Roast in the oven at the same time as the carrots and onion (or immediately after), until the fish is just cooked through, about 10 minutes. Serve atop one of the salads and then garnish with the lemon wedges (if using).

Full recipe: Stir 10 ounces chopped, roasted, chilled turkey or chicken breast plus 1 teaspoon freshly ground black pepper into the salad along with the carrots, onion, and dill in step 3. Alternatively, cut 10 ounces wild Pacific halibut fillets into 4 pieces. Place the 4 pieces onto a 9 × 13-inch baking pan lined with unbleached parchment paper. Brush with 1 tablespoon extra-virgin olive oil and season with 1/8 teaspoon sea salt and 1/8 teaspoon freshly ground black pepper, or to taste. Roast in the oven at the same time as the carrots and onion (or immediately after), until the fish is just cooked through, about 10 minutes. Serve atop each of the salads and then garnish with the lemon wedges (if using).

without
Exchanges/Food Choices: 1 1/2 Starch,
1 Vegetable, 1 Fat
180 calories, 45 calories from fat, 5g total fat,
0.5g saturated fat, 0g trans fat, 0mg cholesterol,
310mg sodium, 210mg potassium, 30g total
carbohydrate, 3g dietary fiber, 2g sugars,
3g protein, 100mg phosphorus

with
Exchanges/Food Choices: 1 1/2 Starch,
1 Vegetable, 3 Lean Meat
300 calories, 70 calories from fat, 8g total fat,
1.5g saturated fat, 0g trans fat, 60mg cholesterol,
370mg sodium, 400mg potassium, 30g total
carbohydrate, 3g dietary fiber, 2g sugars,
25g protein, 260mg phosphorus

Mexican Black Bean Salad

Makes 4 servings: 1 cup each

Juice of 1 lime (2 tablespoons)

1 tablespoon extra-virgin olive oil

1 garlic clove, minced

1/4 teaspoon ground cumin

1/4 teaspoon sea salt, or to taste

1 (15-ounce) can black beans, gently rinsed and drained (1 1/2 cups)

10 cherry tomatoes, sliced, or 20 grape tomatoes, quartered

1 small green bell pepper, diced

1 fresh plum, diced

1/4 cup diced red onion

2 tablespoons chopped fresh cilantro

1 teaspoon finely chopped fresh oregano leaves

1 Hass avocado, pitted, peeled and diced

without

Exchanges/Food Choices: 1 Starch, 1 Vegetable, 2 Fat
200 calories, 80 calories from fat, 9g total fat, 1.5g saturated fat, 0g trans fat, 0mg cholesterol, 270mg sodium, 710mg potassium, 25g total carbohydrate, 7g dietary fiber, 5g sugars, 6g protein, 150mg phosphorus

with

Exchanges/Food Choices: 1 1/2 Starch, 2 Lean Meat, 1 1/2 Fat
260 calories, 100 calories from fat, 12g total fat, 2g saturated fat, 0g trans fat, 25mg cholesterol, 360mg sodium, 820mg potassium, 26g total carbohydrate, 8g dietary fiber, 6g sugars, 15g protein, 220mg phosphorus

Here's a bean and avocado salad that'll appeal to all palates, not just fans of Mexican fare. It packs a punch of flavor, but without the "heat." Providing so many colors, textures, and flavors, it's a real delight. Besides being served as a salad, this recipe can be a cool burrito filling or, if you finely dice the ingredients, a salsa. Consider it a mouthwatering meal multitasker.

1. Whisk together the lime juice, oil, garlic, cumin, and salt in a medium bowl.

2. Add the beans, tomatoes, bell pepper, plum, onion, cilantro, and oregano, and stir until well combined. Let stand for 30 minutes to allow flavors to blend.

3. Gently stir in the avocado, adjust seasoning, and serve in individual bowls.

WITH POULTRY, FISH, OR MEAT

One serving: Grill a 1 1/2-ounce piece of grass-fed beef tenderloin or boneless sirloin until medium-rare, about 2 minutes per side. Sprinkle with a smidgen each of sea salt and chipotle chili powder. Let stand for at least 5 minutes. Cut into about 8 cubes and stir into one of the salads when serving.

Full recipe: Grill a 6-ounce grass-fed beef tenderloin or boneless sirloin steak until medium-rare, about 3 minutes per side. Sprinkle with 1/8 teaspoon each sea salt and chipotle chili powder. Let stand for at least 5 minutes. Cut into about 32 cubes and stir into the salad along with the beans in step 2.

Tropical Banana, Avocado, and Tomato Salad

Makes 4 servings: 2/3 cup each

Don't you love when all you need to do is stir all ingredients together in a bowl? I do—especially when it tastes like you spent a lot of time making the recipe, like this tropical-inspired salad. It's a perfect balance of sweetness and spiciness. Toast whole coriander and cumin seeds and then grind in a coffee grinder or peppermill for an exceptional warm, earthy flair to this cool salad.

Very gently stir together all of the ingredients in a medium bowl, and serve.

{ WITH POULTRY, FISH, OR MEAT }

One serving: Drain 1 1/4 ounces canned no-salt-added, water-packed, white, low-mercury Albacore tuna. Flake into large chunks and stir into 2/3 cup salad along with an additional pinch of sea salt. Arrange the salad in a formed stack on a small plate or serve loosely in a small dish.

Full recipe: Drain one 5-ounce can no-salt-added, water-packed white, low-mercury Albacore tuna. Flake into large chunks and stir into the salad with an additional 1/4 teaspoon sea salt. Arrange the salad in formed stacks on individual plates or serve loosely in 4 small dishes.

1 medium nearly ripe banana (slight amount of green), diced

1 Hass avocado, pitted, peeled, and diced

Juice of 1/2 lime (1 tablespoon)

1 cup grape tomatoes, quartered lengthwise

1 small jalapeño pepper, with half of the seeds, halved lengthwise, very thinly sliced crosswise

1 large garlic clove, minced

1/2 teaspoon ground coriander

1/2 teaspoon ground cumin

1/4 teaspoon sea salt, or to taste

without
Exchanges/Food Choices: 1/2 Fruit, 1 Vegetable, 1 Fat
90 calories, 50 calories from fat, 6g total fat, 1g saturated fat, 0g trans fat, 0mg cholesterol, 150mg sodium, 380mg potassium, 12g total carbohydrate, 4g dietary fiber, 5g sugars, 1g protein, 40mg phosphorus

with
Exchanges/Food Choices: 1/2 Fruit, 1 Vegetable, 1 Lean Meat, 1 Fat
140 calories, 60 calories from fat, 7g total fat, 1g saturated fat, 0g trans fat, 15mg cholesterol, 310mg sodium, 460mg potassium, 12g total carbohydrate, 4g dietary fiber, 5g sugars, 10g protein, 110mg phosphorus

CHAPTER 4

soups, stews, and chilis

Red Onion Soup with Shiitake Broth

Makes 5 servings: 1 cup each

2 teaspoons canola or grapeseed oil

3 large red onions, halved and thinly sliced

2 teaspoons white balsamic or white wine vinegar

1/2 teaspoon + 1/8 teaspoon sea salt, or to taste

1 cup fresh thinly sliced shiitake mushrooms, stems removed

1 (32-fluid ounce) carton low-sodium vegetable broth

1/2 teaspoon freshly ground black pepper, or to taste

1 1/2 teaspoons minced fresh rosemary

1 teaspoon finely chopped fresh thyme leaves + 5 fresh thyme sprigs

10 whole-grain pita chips

1/4 cup shredded Gruyère or other aged Swiss cheese (1 ounce)

I got hooked on French onion soup after I was lucky enough to slurp a bowl of it in France. I wanted to enjoy it at home in a more healthful way, so I created a hearty, onion-loaded, mushroom broth–based version that doesn't need to be laden with cheese. The umami ("meaty" taste) from the shiitakes creates such a savory broth that you'll find this recipe to be more enjoyable than the cheesy, beef broth–based original.

1. Heat the oil in a nonstick stockpot or extra-large saucepan over medium heat. Add the onions, vinegar, and 1/8 teaspoon salt, and cook while stirring occasionally until softened, about 10 minutes. Increase heat to medium-high, add the mushrooms, and sauté until the onions are well caramelized, about 15 minutes. Add the broth, the remaining 1/2 teaspoon salt, the pepper, rosemary, and the chopped thyme, and bring to a boil over high heat. Reduce heat to low, cover, and simmer until the flavors are developed, about 10 minutes. Meanwhile, preheat the oven to 500°F.

2. Place 5 ovenproof soup bowls or crocks onto a baking sheet. Adjust seasoning and ladle the soup into each bowl. Place 2 pita chips on top of each and sprinkle with the cheese. Bake in the oven on the top oven rack until the cheese is bubbly, about 4 minutes.

3. Garnish each with a thyme sprig, and serve.

WITH POULTRY, FISH, OR MEAT

One serving: Cut 1/2 ounce lean, uncured ham into matchstick-size strips. Place into one of the bowls before ladling in the soup in step 2. Garnish with a few of the matchstick-size ham strips instead of or in addition to a thyme sprig, if desired.

Full recipe: Cut 2 1/2 ounces lean, uncured ham into matchstick-size strips. Place into the bowls before ladling in the soup in step 2. Garnish each with a few of the matchstick-size ham strips instead of or in addition to the thyme sprigs, if desired.

without
Exchanges/Food Choices: 1 Carbohydrate, 1 Fat
110 calories, 45 calories from fat, 5g total fat,
1.3g saturated fat, 0g trans fat,
5mg cholesterol, 370mg sodium,
190mg potassium, 13g total carbohydrate, 2g
dietary fiber, 4g sugars, 4g protein,
80mg phosphorus

with
Exchanges/Food Choices: 1 Carbohydrate,
1 Lean Meat, 1 Fat
120 calories, 45 calories from fat, 5g total fat,
1.5g saturated fat, 0g trans fat,
15mg cholesterol, 460mg sodium,
230mg potassium, 13g total carbohydrate,
2g dietary fiber, 5g sugars, 7g protein,
110mg phosphorus

Spanish Roasted Tomato Soup with Chèvre

Makes 8 servings: 1 cup each

2 pounds plum tomatoes, quartered lengthwise

4 large garlic cloves, unpeeled

1 tablespoon extra-virgin olive oil

1 medium red onion, finely diced

1 tablespoon aged balsamic vinegar

1 teaspoon sea salt, divided

1 1/2 teaspoons finely chopped fresh rosemary + 8 small rosemary sprigs

1 teaspoon chopped fresh oregano leaves (optional)

3/4 teaspoon freshly ground black pepper, or to taste

Pinch ground cayenne pepper or smoked paprika

6 cups low-sodium vegetable broth

2 tablespoons crumbled chèvre (soft goat cheese)

Whoa! This soup is brilliantly full-flavored. The tomatoes are roasted, which adds so much depth to the recipe. And the blending of herbs and spices creates a fragrant marriage of flavor. The sprinkling of goat cheese is the ideal tangy, creamy, finishing accent. It's a true showstopper for your taste buds.

1. Preheat the oven to 375°F. Spread the tomatoes, skin side down, and garlic on a large baking sheet. Roast until the tomatoes are very soft and their skin is caramelized, about 45 minutes, while removing the garlic about halfway through the roasting. Set aside.

2. Heat the oil in a stockpot or Dutch oven over medium-high heat. Add the onion, vinegar, and 1/4 teaspoon salt, and sauté until the onion is slightly caramelized, about 8 minutes.

3. Add the tomatoes, garlic cloves (squeezed out of their skin), chopped rosemary, oregano (if using), black pepper, cayenne, broth, and the remaining 3/4 teaspoon salt. Increase heat to high and bring to a boil. Reduce heat to medium-low and simmer, uncovered, to allow flavors to blend and soup to reduce, about 30 minutes. Remove from the heat and purée to a slightly textured consistency using a handheld immersion blender. Adjust seasoning.

4. Ladle the soup into individual bowls, sprinkle with the chèvre, and serve.

One serving: Place 2 small mussels in a small saucepan along with 1 tablespoon unsweetened green tea or water. Sprinkle with about 1 tablespoon finely diced red onion and 1 minced small garlic clove. Cover and place over high heat until the mussels open. Serve the mussels on top of one bowl of soup instead of the chèvre in step 4. Sprinkle with 1/2 teaspoon extra-virgin olive oil and a smidgen of minced fresh rosemary. Alternatively, place 3 small precooked chicken meatballs in the center of one of the bowls before ladling in the soup.

Full recipe: Fill a pot with 16 small mussels and add 1/2 cup unsweetened green tea or water. Sprinkle with 1/2 cup chopped red onion and 2 minced large garlic cloves. Cover and place over high heat until the mussels open. Discard any that do not open. Serve 2 mussels on top of each bowl of soup instead of the chèvre in step 4. Sprinkle each with 1/2 teaspoon extra-virgin olive oil and a smidgen of minced fresh rosemary. Alternatively, place 3 small precooked chicken meatballs in the center of each of the bowls before ladling in the soup.

without
Exchanges/Food Choices: 1 Vegetable, 1/2 Fat
60 calories, 20 calories from fat, 2.5g total fat, 0.5g saturated fat, 0g trans fat, 0mg cholesterol, 410mg sodium, 280mg potassium, 8g total carbohydrate, 2g dietary fiber, 5g sugars, 1g protein, 30mg phosphorus

with
Exchanges/Food Choices: 1 Vegetable, 1/2 Lean Meat, 1 Fat
90 calories, 40 calories from fat, 5g total fat, 0.5g saturated fat, 0g trans fat, 5mg cholesterol, 460mg sodium, 360mg potassium, 10g total carbohydrate, 2g dietary fiber, 5g sugars, 4g protein, 70mg phosphorus

Caramelized Butternut Squash Potage

Makes 8 servings: 1 cup each

1 tablespoon extra-virgin olive oil

1 large white onion or sweet onion, chopped

2 teaspoons apple cider vinegar

3/4 teaspoon + 1/8 teaspoon sea salt, or to taste

3 cups cubed butternut squash (1 pound)

1 1/2 cups chopped cauliflower florets

1 large garlic clove, minced

1 (32-fluid ounce) carton low-sodium vegetable broth

3/4 teaspoon freshly ground black pepper, or to taste

1/4 teaspoon ground sage, or to taste

1/8 teaspoon ground cayenne pepper, or to taste

1 (12-fluid ounce) can fat-free evaporated milk

6 fresh sage leaves (optional)

After the bounty of summer produce, butternut is a winter squash, which becomes a standout, and a standby, for rustic dishes. One of my favorite ways to enjoy it is in a cozy cup of soup, like this steamy, slightly creamy recipe. It's full of comfort and sweet savoriness along with a pleasant kick. The sage adds flavor intrigue.

1. Heat the oil in a nonstick Dutch oven over medium-high heat. Add the onion, vinegar, and 1/8 teaspoon salt, and sauté until the onion is softened, about 5 minutes. Add the squash and cauliflower, and sauté until all vegetables are lightly caramelized, about 7 minutes. Add the garlic and sauté for 30 seconds.

2. Stir in the broth, 1 cup water, pepper, sage, cayenne, and the remaining 3/4 teaspoon salt, and bring to a boil over high heat. Reduce heat to low and simmer, covered, until the squash is tender, stirring a couple times, about 28 minutes. Stir in the evaporated milk and simmer uncovered for 5 minutes.

3. Remove from the heat. Purée until smooth using a handheld immersion blender. If desired, continue to simmer to desired reduced consistency. Adjust seasoning.

4. Ladle into individual bowls, garnish each with a sage leaf (if using), and serve.

{ WITH POULTRY, FISH, OR MEAT }

One serving: Sprinkle 1 ounce shredded rotisserie chicken, white or dark meat, with a smidgen of freshly ground black pepper. After puréeing the soup in step 3, transfer 1 cup soup to a small saucepan. Add the seasoned chicken and simmer for 5 minutes. Ladle into a bowl and garnish with a sage leaf, if desired.

Full recipe: Sprinkle 8 ounces shredded rotisserie chicken, white or dark meat, with 1/4 teaspoon freshly ground black pepper. After puréeing the soup in step 3, stir in the seasoned chicken and simmer for 5 minutes. Ladle into individual bowls and garnish each with a sage leaf, if desired.

without
Exchanges/Food Choices: 1 Carbohydrate, 1/2 Fat
90 calories, 15 calories from fat, 2g total fat,
0g saturated fat, 0g trans fat, 0mg cholesterol,
380mg sodium, 350mg potassium, 15g total
carbohydrate, 3g dietary fiber, 9g sugars,
5g protein, 120mg phosphorus

with
Exchanges/Food Choices: 1 Carbohydrate,
1 Lean Meat, 1/2 Fat
130 calories, 25 calories from fat, 3g total fat,
0.5g saturated fat, 0g trans fat, 25mg cholesterol,
480mg sodium, 440mg potassium, 15g total
carbohydrate, 3g dietary fiber, 9g sugars,
13g protein, 190mg phosphorus

Gingery Asparagus, Couscous, and Crimini Soup

Makes 8 servings: 1 cup each

1 1/2 teaspoons grapeseed or
    canola oil

1 teaspoon toasted sesame oil

1 medium yellow onion, diced

1 tablespoon brown rice vinegar,
    divided

1/2 teaspoon sea salt, divided

1/4 teaspoon dried hot pepper flakes,
    or to taste

2 large garlic cloves, minced

1 1/2 tablespoons freshly grated
    gingerroot

3 scallions, thinly sliced, green and
    white parts separated

5 cups low-sodium vegetable broth

1 tablespoon + 2 teaspoons naturally
    brewed soy sauce, or to taste

1 pound asparagus, trimmed, cut into
    3/4-inch pieces on the diagonal

1 (8-ounce) package crimini
    mushrooms, sliced

2/3 cup whole-wheat couscous

Attention ginger lovers! This soup is especially designed for you. Though I hope everyone gives it a try. It's as delicious day two as it is day one. The leftovers are great after the flavors have time to mingle; simply reheat in the microwave. Plus, the ginger in it may actually help to alleviate tummy woes.

1. Heat the oils in a stockpot or Dutch oven over medium-high heat. Add the onion, 1 teaspoon vinegar, 1/4 teaspoon of the salt, and the hot pepper flakes, and sauté until the onion is lightly caramelized, about 8 minutes. Add the garlic, ginger, and white part of the scallions, and sauté for 30 seconds.

2. Add the broth, soy sauce, and the remaining 2 teaspoons vinegar and 1/4 teaspoon salt, and bring to a boil over high heat. Stir in the asparagus and mushrooms. Cover and simmer over low heat until the asparagus is nearly tender, about 10 minutes. Stir in the couscous, cover, and simmer until the couscous is fully cooked, about 5 minutes. Stir in about three-fourths of the green part of the scallions, and adjust seasoning.

3. Ladle into individual bowls, sprinkle with the remaining green part of the scallions, and serve. Serve with additional soy sauce on the side, if desired.

{ WITH POULTRY, FISH, OR MEAT }

One serving: Shred 1 ounce roasted chicken thigh, or separate premium, picked-over, wild claw lump crabmeat into chunks. Add to one of the bowls before ladling in the soup.

Full recipe: Shred 8 ounces roasted chicken thigh, or separate premium, picked-over, wild claw lump crabmeat into chunks. Stir into the soup along with the scallions in step 2.

without
Exchanges/Food Choices: 1 Starch, 1 Vegetable
100 calories, 15 calories from fat, 1.5g total fat, 0g saturated fat, 0g trans fat, 0mg cholesterol, 430mg sodium, 260mg potassium, 19g total carbohydrate, 4g dietary fiber, 3g sugars, 4g protein, 80mg phosphorus

with
Exchanges/Food Choices: 1 Starch, 1 Vegetable, 1 Lean Meat, 1/2 Fat
150 calories, 35 calories from fat, 4g total fat, 1g saturated fat, 0g trans fat, 40mg cholesterol, 460mg sodium, 340mg potassium, 19g total carbohydrate, 4g dietary fiber, 3g sugars, 11g protein, 140mg phosphorus

How to Store Fresh Gingerroot

Extending the shelf life of gingerroot starts at the market. Choose pieces that are firm and fragrant. No mushy stuff! If you have more than you need, just freeze unused ginger in an airtight container for up to six months. When you're ready to use it, simply grate it in its frozen state.

Szechuan Veggie Dumpling Soup

Makes 4 servings: 1 2/3 cups each

2 teaspoons grapeseed or canola oil

2 teaspoons toasted sesame oil

4 scallions, thinly sliced, green and white parts separated

2 large garlic cloves, thinly sliced

2 teaspoons freshly grated gingerroot

2 teaspoons brown rice vinegar

1 (32-fluid ounce) carton low-sodium vegetable broth

1/4 cup freshly squeezed orange juice

1 1/2 teaspoons naturally brewed soy sauce, or to taste

2 bunches fresh baby bok choy, thinly sliced

1 medium red or orange bell pepper, thinly sliced

1/2 cup snow peas, very thinly sliced

1/4 teaspoon dried hot pepper flakes, or to taste

12 frozen whole-grain vegetarian dumplings or Steamed Edamame Dumplings (page 50)

1 teaspoon white or black sesame seeds, toasted

There's no need to get Chinese takeout now that you can make this flavorsome Asian-inspired soup yourself. The dumplings make it fun and filling; plus, you can purchase frozen dumplings to simplify the recipe. Hint: If you're preparing both the veggie and meat versions, use black sesame seeds for topping the veggie version and white for topping the meat version, so you'll know the difference.

1. Heat the oils in a large saucepan over medium-high heat. Add the white part of the scallions, the garlic, ginger, and vinegar, and sauté until the scallions are softened, about 1 1/2 minutes. Add the broth, orange juice, soy sauce, bok choy, bell pepper, snow peas, the green part of the scallions, and the hot pepper flakes, and bring just to a boil over high heat. Reduce heat to medium, cover, and simmer until the bok choy is crisp-tender, about 5 minutes.

2. Add the frozen dumplings, cover, and simmer until the dumplings are cooked through, about 8 minutes. Adjust seasoning.

3. Ladle into individual bowls and sprinkle with the sesame seeds. If desired, garnish with additional sliced scallions, and serve with additional soy sauce on the side.

{ WITH POULTRY, FISH, OR MEAT }

One serving: Before adding the dumplings in step 2, transfer 1 1/4 cups (one serving without dumplings) of the soup to a small saucepan. Add 3 frozen whole-grain shrimp dumplings or chicken dumplings (or the meat version of Steamed Edamame Dumplings; page 51) to the small saucepan. Add only 9 vegetarian dumplings to the large saucepan. Simmer until the dumplings are cooked through.

Full recipe: In step 2, add 12 frozen whole-grain shrimp dumplings or chicken dumplings (or the meat version of Steamed Edamame Dumplings; page 51) to the soup instead of the vegetarian dumplings.

without
Exchanges/Food Choices: 1 Starch, 1 Vegetable, 2 Fat
180 calories, 70 calories from fat, 8g total fat, 1g saturated fat, 0g trans fat, 0mg cholesterol, 410mg sodium, 460mg potassium, 22g total carbohydrate, 4g dietary fiber, 8g sugars, 6g protein, 80mg phosphorus

with
Exchanges/Food Choices: 1 Starch, 1 Vegetable, 1 Lean Meat, 1 Fat
220 calories, 70 calories from fat, 8g total fat, 1g saturated fat, 0g trans fat, 10mg cholesterol, 600mg sodium, 550mg potassium, 27g total carbohydrate, 4g dietary fiber, 8g sugars, 12g protein, 220mg phosphorus

Beech and Summer Squash Soba Bowl

Makes 6 servings: 1 1/2 cups each

1 tablespoon unrefined peanut or
canola oil

1 large white onion, finely diced

Juice of 1 lime (2 tablespoons),
divided + 1 lime cut into 6 wedges

1/2 teaspoon sea salt, divided

1 tablespoon freshly grated gingerroot

2 large garlic cloves, minced

6 cups low-sodium vegetable broth

2 medium yellow summer squash
or zucchini, unpeeled, halved
lengthwise and thinly sliced
crosswise

1 (2.5-ounce) package beech
mushrooms, separated, or oyster
mushrooms

1 1/4 teaspoons naturally brewed soy
sauce, or to taste

1/2 teaspoon freshly ground black
pepper, or to taste

5 ounces buckwheat soba noodles or
whole-grain udon noodles

1/3 cup chopped fresh cilantro

Soup isn't only intended to be slurped down in winter. Here's a gingery soup that's designed for summertime (and beyond) as it's made with summer squash. It's full of soba noodles, too, which make this soup so satisfying that you can serve it as an entrée, if you like. The cilantro is the tasty finish that ties everything together.

1. Heat the oil in a stockpot or Dutch oven over medium heat. Add the onion, 1 tablespoon lime juice, and 1/4 teaspoon salt, and sauté until the onion is fully softened, about 10 minutes. Add the ginger and garlic, and sauté for 2 minutes. Add the broth, summer squash, mushrooms, soy sauce, pepper, and the remaining 1/4 teaspoon salt, and bring to a full boil over high heat. Stir in the noodles, reduce heat to medium-low, and simmer, uncovered, until the summer squash and noodles are just softened, about 6 minutes. Stir in the remaining lime juice. Adjust seasoning.

2. Ladle the soup into individual bowls, sprinkle with the cilantro, garnish with the lime wedges, and enjoy with chopsticks and a spoon. Serve with additional soy sauce on the side, if desired.

{ WITH POULTRY, FISH, OR MEAT }

One serving: Add 1 minced scallion, green and white parts, 1/4 teaspoon freshly grated gingerroot, and 1/4 teaspoon naturally brewed soy sauce (if desired) to 1 1/2 ounces ground turkey (about 94% lean). Combine and form into 5 mini-meatballs. (Note: The meatballs will be very soft but will firm upon cooking.) Heat 1/2 teaspoon canola oil in a small, nonstick skillet over medium-high heat. Add the meatballs and gently sauté until browned and well done, about 5 minutes. Add 4 of the meatballs to one of the soup bowls, then ladle in the soup in step 2 and top with the remaining meatball.

Full recipe: Add 6 minced scallions, green and white parts, 1 1/2 teaspoons freshly grated gingerroot, and 1 1/2 teaspoons naturally brewed soy sauce (if desired) to 9 ounces of ground turkey (about 94% lean). Combine and form into 30 mini-meatballs. (Note: The meatballs will be very soft but will firm upon cooking.) Heat 1 tablespoon canola oil in a large, nonstick skillet over medium-high heat. Add the meatballs and gently sauté until browned and well done, about 5 minutes. Prepare in two batches, if necessary. Stir the meatballs into the soup in step 1 just before adding the noodles.

without
Exchanges/Food Choices: 1/2 Starch, 1 Vegetable, 1/2 Fat
150 calories, 20 calories from fat, 2.5g total fat, 0.5g saturated fat, 0g trans fat, 0mg cholesterol, 460mg sodium, 270mg potassium, 28g total carbohydrate, 2g dietary fiber, 5g sugars, 6g protein, 60mg phosphorus

with
Exchanges/Food Choices: 1 Starch, 1 Vegetable, 1 Lean Meat, 1 Fat
240 calories, 80 calories from fat, 9g total fat, 1.5g saturated fat, 0g trans fat, 30mg cholesterol, 490mg sodium, 400mg potassium, 29g total carbohydrate, 3g dietary fiber, 5g sugars, 14g protein, 150mg phosphorus

A Hint of "Heat"

A key ingredient in soup is salt. It's basically what helps make soup taste like soup. When you're trying to keep your total daily intake of sodium to a minimum, consider adding a hint of "heat" to provide more flavor depth. Splash your soup serving with a few drops of hot pepper sauce. Or consider global flair by using curry paste or harissa. Try this: stir 1/2 teaspoon green curry paste into the Beech and Summer Squash Soba Bowl recipe.

Black Bean, Poblano, and Tortilla Soup

Makes 6 servings: 1 cup each

2 teaspoons unrefined peanut or
   canola oil

1 medium Poblano pepper, finely diced

1 small or 1/2 large white onion, finely
   diced

Juice and zest of 1 lime
   (2 tablespoons juice), divided

1/2 teaspoon sea salt, divided

1 small jalapeño pepper, with some
   seeds, minced

2 large garlic cloves, minced

1 (32-fluid ounce) carton low-sodium
   vegetable broth

1 (15-ounce) can no-salt-added black
   beans, drained (1 1/2 cups)

1 (14.5-ounce) can crushed roasted
   tomatoes (1 3/4 cups)

1 teaspoon finely chopped fresh
   oregano leaves

1/4 teaspoon ground cumin

1/4 cup chopped fresh cilantro

12 unsalted yellow or white corn
   tortilla chips, coarsely broken

1 Hass avocado, pitted, peeled, diced

If you're a Mexican cuisine aficionada or aficionado, this high-flavored, tomato-based soup should be at the top of your list. The black beans make it exceptionally satisfying and extra nutritious. And the crisp tortilla chip and creamy avocado topping make it festive.

1. Heat the oil in a stockpot or Dutch oven over medium-high heat. Add the Poblano pepper, onion, 2 teaspoons lime juice, and 1/4 teaspoon salt, and sauté until the onion is lightly caramelized, about 8 minutes. Add the jalapeño and garlic, and sauté for 1 minute. Add the broth, beans, tomatoes, oregano, cumin, and the remaining 1/4 teaspoon salt, and bring to a boil over high heat. Reduce heat to medium and simmer, uncovered, until the Poblano peppers are fully softened, about 15 minutes.

2. Remove from heat. Stir in the cilantro and the remaining lime juice. Adjust seasoning.

3. Ladle into bowls, top with tortilla chips, avocado, and desired amount of the lime zest, and serve.

{ WITH POULTRY, FISH, OR MEAT }

One serving: Add 1 tablespoon medium salsa drained of excess liquid and 1 unsalted, finely crushed yellow corn tortilla chip to 1 1/2 ounces ground turkey (about 94% lean) or ground chicken breast. Combine and form into 5 mini-meatballs. (Note: The meatballs will be very soft but will firm upon cooking.) Heat 1/2 teaspoon canola or grapeseed oil in a small, nonstick skillet over medium-high heat. Add the meatballs and gently sauté until browned and well done, about 5 minutes. Add to one of the bowls before ladling in the soup in step 3.

Full recipe: Add 6 tablespoons medium salsa drained of excess liquid and 6 unsalted, finely crushed yellow corn tortilla chips to 9 ounces ground turkey (about 94% lean) or ground chicken breast. Combine and form into 30 mini-meatballs. (Note: The meatballs will be very soft but will firm upon cooking.) Heat 1 tablespoon canola or grapeseed oil in a large, nonstick skillet over medium-high heat. Add the meatballs and gently sauté until browned and well done, about 5 minutes. Prepare in two batches, if necessary. Stir the meatballs into the soup in step 1 after the soup comes to a boil.

without
Exchanges/Food Choices: 1 Starch, 1 1/2 Vegetable, 1 Fat
170 calories, 60 calories from fat, 6g total fat, 1g saturated fat, 0g trans fat, 0mg cholesterol, 390mg sodium, 540mg potassium, 25g total carbohydrate, 8g dietary fiber, 5g sugars, 6g protein, 110mg phosphorus

with
Exchanges/Food Choices: 1 Starch, 1 Vegetable, 1 Lean Meat, 2 Fat
270 calories, 120 calories from fat, 13g total fat, 2.3g saturated fat, 0g trans fat, 30mg cholesterol, 420mg sodium, 630mg potassium, 26g total carbohydrate, 8g dietary fiber, 5g sugars, 14g protein, 200mg phosphorus

Creamy Herbed White Bean Soup

Makes 5 servings: 1 cup each

2 teaspoons extra-virgin olive oil

1 large white onion, finely chopped

Juice of 1 small lemon
(2 tablespoons), divided

1/2 teaspoon sea salt, divided

1 large garlic clove, minced

1 (32-fluid ounce) carton low-sodium
vegetable broth

1 (15-ounce) can no-salt-added
cannellini or butter beans, drained
(1 1/2 cups)

1/2 teaspoon freshly ground black
pepper, or to taste

1 teaspoon minced fresh rosemary
or dill

1 teaspoon chopped fresh chives
or dill

Comfort food can taste luxurious. This puréed cannellini bean soup proves it. You'll especially love the fresh rosemary accent, which makes the soup come alive. If your aim is to make this soup family-friendly, serve it along with a small handful of whole-grain pita chips for dipping into its creamy goodness.

1. Heat the oil in a large saucepan over medium heat. Add the onion, 1 tablespoon lemon juice, and 1/4 teaspoon salt, and sauté until the onion is softened, about 8 minutes. Add the garlic and sauté for 1 minute.

2. Add the broth, beans, pepper, and the remaining 1 tablespoon lemon juice and 1/4 teaspoon salt. Bring to a boil over high heat. Reduce the heat to medium-low and simmer, covered, until the onion and beans are fully softened, about 20 minutes.

3. Purée in a blender in batches using the hot fill line as a guide. Return to a saucepan over medium-low heat. Stir in the rosemary. Adjust seasoning.

4. Ladle into individual bowls, sprinkle with the chives, and serve.

{ WITH POULTRY, FISH, OR MEAT }

One serving: Prepare 1/2 ounce fully cooked sweet Italian poultry sausage link according to package directions. Slice the sausage very thin and sprinkle onto one of the soups before the chives in step 4.

Full recipe: Prepare 2 1/2 ounces fully cooked sweet Italian poultry sausage link according to package directions. Slice the sausage very thin and sprinkle onto each of the soups before the chives in step 4.

without
Exchanges/Food Choices: 1 Starch, 1 Vegetable, 1/2 Fat
110 calories, 20 calories from fat, 2.5g total fat, 0g saturated fat, 0g trans fat, 0mg cholesterol, 370mg sodium, 220mg potassium, 17g total carbohydrate, 5g dietary fiber, 4g sugars, 4g protein, 80mg phosphorus

with
Exchanges/Food Choices: 1 Starch, 1/2 Vegetable, 1 Lean Meat
130 calories, 35 calories from fat, 4g total fat, 0.5g saturated fat, 0g trans fat, 10mg cholesterol, 460mg sodium, 250mg potassium, 17g total carbohydrate, 5g dietary fiber, 4g sugars, 7g protein, 100mg phosphorus

Rustic Vegetable Stew

1 tablespoon extra-virgin olive oil

1 jumbo yellow or red onion, quartered and thinly sliced

Juice of 1 lemon (3 tablespoons), divided

1/4 teaspoon + 1/8 teaspoon sea salt, or to taste

3 large garlic cloves, minced

1 (28-ounce) can crushed roasted tomatoes

1 (32-fluid ounce) carton low-sodium vegetable broth

3 tablespoons hummus of choice (page 59)

2 cups fresh green beans, ends trimmed, cut in half on the diagonal

2 cups small baby carrots

8 ounces blue or Dutch yellow baby potatoes, halved

2 large celery stalks, cut into 1/2-inch slices on the diagonal

1 teaspoon freshly ground black pepper, or to taste

2 tablespoons finely chopped fresh tarragon or basil, divided

The veggies in this bowl of rustic goodness are hearty and plentiful. But it's what you don't see that's creating extra body—hummus is the surprise ingredient. Savor every spoonful of this stew slowly to soothe your soul and please your palate.

1. Heat the oil in a stockpot over medium-high heat. Add the onion, 1 tablespoon lemon juice, and 1/4 teaspoon salt, and sauté until the onion is softened and lightly caramelized, about 8 minutes. Add the garlic and sauté for 30 seconds.

2. Add the tomatoes, broth, hummus, green beans, carrots, potatoes, celery, pepper, and the remaining lemon juice and 1/8 teaspoon salt, and bring to a boil over high heat. Reduce heat to low, cover, and simmer until all the vegetables are fully cooked, about 40 minutes. Stir in 1 tablespoon tarragon. Adjust seasoning.

3. Ladle into individual bowls, sprinkle with the remaining 1 tablespoon tarragon, and serve.

{ WITH POULTRY, FISH, OR MEAT }

One serving: After the stew has been simmering for 30 minutes, transfer 1 1/4 cups to a small saucepan and add 1 ounce shredded or cubed rotisserie or roasted chicken thigh. Simmer, covered, for 10 minutes. Ladle into a bowl, garnish with tarragon, and serve.

Full recipe: After the stew has been simmering for about 30 minutes, add 8 ounces shredded or cubed rotisserie or roasted chicken thigh. Continue to simmer for 10 minutes more.

without
Exchanges/Food Choices: 3 Vegetable, 1/2 Fat
120 calories, 25 calories from fat, 3g total fat, 0g saturated fat, 0g trans fat, 0mg cholesterol, 370mg sodium, 640mg potassium, 22g total carbohydrate, 6g dietary fiber, 9g sugars, 4g protein, 90mg phosphorus

with
Exchanges/Food Choices: 3 Vegetable, 1 Lean Meat, 1 Fat
180 calories, 50 calories from fat, 6g total fat, 1g saturated fat, 0g trans fat, 35mg cholesterol, 470mg sodium, 710mg potassium, 22g total carbohydrate, 6g dietary fiber, 9g sugars, 11g protein, 150mg phosphorus

Indian Sweet Potato-Edamame Stew

Makes 5 servings: 1 2/3 cups each

2 teaspoons extra-virgin olive oil

1 large white onion, cut into large dices

2 large garlic cloves, minced

1 teaspoon harissa or 1/4 teaspoon hot pepper sauce, or to taste

3/4 teaspoon ground cinnamon

3/4 teaspoon ground coriander

1 (15-ounce) can diced tomatoes (with liquid)

3 medium-large (9-ounce) sweet potatoes, unpeeled, root ends trimmed, cut into 1-inch cubes (8 cups cubes)

2 cups low-sodium vegetable broth

1/2 teaspoon freshly ground black pepper, or to taste

1 1/2 cups thawed frozen shelled edamame

1/2 teaspoon sea salt, or to taste

1/4 cup roughly chopped fresh cilantro, or to taste

Love Indian food? You'll be enamored with this entrée-size stew. Haven't yet become an Indian cuisine enthusiast? This inspired stew is a scrumptious starting point. The cinnamon and coriander provide a just-right worldly accent to the large bites of sweet potatoes and the unique addition of edamame. The cilantro goes beyond a regular garnish and adds freshness at serving time.

1. Heat the oil in a stockpot or Dutch oven over medium-high heat. Add the onion and sauté until lightly caramelized, about 8 minutes. Add the garlic, harissa, cinnamon, and coriander, and sauté for 30 seconds. Add the tomatoes with liquid, sweet potatoes, broth, and black pepper, and bring to a boil over high heat. Reduce heat to low, cover, and simmer until the sweet potatoes are cooked through and softened, about 45 minutes.

2. Stir in the edamame and salt and continue to simmer, covered, until the edamame is fully heated, about 10 minutes. Add salt to taste.

3. Ladle the stew into individual bowls, sprinkle with the cilantro, and serve.

{ WITH POULTRY, FISH, OR MEAT }

One serving: After adding the edamame and before adding salt, ladle 1 2/3 cups stew from step 2 into a small saucepan. Stir in 1 fully cooked rotisserie chicken drumstick with skin or 3 homemade or packaged fully cooked whole-grain chicken nuggets, like the chicken version of Oven-Fried Nuggets (skip the marinara; page 47), into a small saucepan. Cover and simmer over low heat until the chicken is heated through and absorbs some of the stew, about 10 minutes. Adjust seasoning.

Full recipe: Add 5 fully cooked rotisserie chicken drumsticks with skin or 15 homemade or packaged fully cooked whole-grain chicken nuggets, like the chicken version of Oven-Fried Nuggets (skip the marinara; page 47), into the stew along with the sweet potatoes in step 1. Skip the salt in step 2.

without
Exchanges/Food Choices: 2 Starch,
1 1/2 Vegetable, 1 Lean Meat
250 calories, 40 calories from fat, 4.5g total fat,
0.5g saturated fat, 0g trans fat, 0mg cholesterol,
570mg sodium, 770mg potassium, 44g total
carbohydrate, 9g dietary fiber, 12g sugars,
9g protein, 160mg phosphorus

with
Exchanges/Food Choices: 2 Starch,
1 1/2 Vegetable, 2 Medium-Fat Meat, 1 Fat
360 calories, 100 calories from fat, 11g total fat,
2g saturated fat, 0g trans fat, 85mg cholesterol,
550mg sodium, 930mg potassium, 44g total
carbohydrate, 9g dietary fiber, 12g sugars,
23g protein, 300mg phosphorus

Roasted "Baba Ghanoush" Stew

Makes 6 servings: 1 rounded cup stew each

1 large (1 1/2-pound) eggplant, unpeeled

2 teaspoons extra-virgin olive oil

1 medium yellow or white onion, diced

2 large garlic cloves, thinly sliced

1 (32-fluid ounce) carton low-sodium vegetable broth

Juice of 1 lemon (3 tablespoons)

2 tablespoons tahini

3/4 teaspoon sea salt, or to taste

1/4 teaspoon ground cumin

1/2 cup chopped fresh flat-leaf parsley, divided

1 large whole-wheat or other whole-grain pita, toasted, broken into small bite-size pieces

Baba ghanoush is a Middle Eastern roasted eggplant dip. Every ingredient in the dip is found in this reinvented, earthy stew. And instead of dipping pita into dip, you'll be stirring bite-size pieces of toasted pita into the stew. Serve it as an appetizer. If you prefer the meat version, consider it an entrée.

1. Preheat the oven to 450°F. Prick the eggplant several times with a fork. Roast the eggplant (do not wrap in foil) on a baking pan lined with unbleached parchment paper until fully cooked, about 35 minutes. Let cool slightly. Cut into 3/4–1-inch cubes (do not peel) and discard stem.

2. Heat the oil in a large saucepan over medium-high heat. Add the onion and sauté for 1 minute; add the garlic and sauté for 1 minute. Add the eggplant cubes, broth, lemon juice, tahini, salt, cumin, and 1/4 cup parsley, and bring to a full boil over high heat. Reduce heat to medium-low, cover, and simmer until stew-like, about 45 minutes. Stir in the pita pieces, cover, and simmer until the bread is fully softened, about 5 minutes more. Adjust seasoning.

3. Ladle the stew into individual bowls. Sprinkle with the remaining 1/4 cup parsley, and serve.

{ WITH POULTRY, FISH, OR MEAT }

One serving: Heat 1/2 teaspoon extra-virgin olive oil in a small, nonstick skillet over medium-high heat. Add 1 1/2 ounces lean ground lamb or beef sirloin and sauté until crumbled and browned, about 1 1/2 minutes. Season with about a pinch each of sea salt, freshly ground black pepper, and ground cinnamon. Sprinkle onto one of the bowls of stew before the parsley in step 3.

Full recipe: Heat 1 tablespoon extra-virgin olive oil in a large, nonstick skillet over medium-high heat. Add 9 ounces lean ground lamb or beef sirloin and sauté until crumbled and browned, about 2 minutes. Season with 1/4 teaspoon each sea salt, freshly ground black pepper, and ground cinnamon. Divide evenly atop the stew before sprinkling with the parsley in step 3.

without
Exchanges/Food Choices: 1/2 Starch,
1 1/2 Vegetable,1 Fat
120 calories, 45 calories from fat, 5g total fat,
0.5g saturated fat, 0g trans fat, 0mg cholesterol,
440mg sodium, 370mg potassium, 19g total
carbohydrate, 6g dietary fiber, 6g sugars,
3g protein, 90mg phosphorus

with
Exchanges/Food Choices: 1/2 Starch,
1 1/2 Vegetable, 1 Lean Meat, 1 1/2 Fat
190 calories, 80 calories from fat, 9g total fat,
2g saturated fat, 0g trans fat, 20mg cholesterol,
560mg sodium, 450mg potassium, 19g total
carbohydrate, 6g dietary fiber, 6g sugars,
10g protein, 150mg phosphorus

Garlic Spinach Dal Stew

Makes 6 servings: 1 cup each

2 teaspoons extra-virgin olive oil

1 medium red onion, diced

2 large celery stalks, diced

1 small Serrano pepper, with seeds, minced

Juice and zest of 1 lemon (3 tablespoons juice)

3/4 teaspoons sea salt, divided

3 large garlic cloves, thinly sliced or minced

5 cups low-sodium vegetable broth

3/4 cup dried French green lentils, rinsed and drained

1 pint grape tomatoes

1/2 teaspoon + 1/8 teaspoon South Asian Spice Trio (page 129)

1/2 teaspoon freshly ground black pepper, or to taste

5 cups packed fresh baby spinach (5 ounces)

1/4 cup plain fat-free Greek yogurt (optional)

"Dal" refers to legumes, like lentils. It also refers to a soup or other dish made with them, like this tangy, lentil-based stew. Its rich South Asian goodness—with a spice trio of cumin, coriander, and turmeric—will tingle your taste buds. And the pops of color and flavor from the grape tomatoes and fresh baby spinach create more appeal. In fact, try this stew around the winter holidays when those pops of red and green provide festive delight.

1. Heat the oil in a stockpot over medium-high heat. Add the onion, celery, Serrano pepper, lemon juice, and 1/4 teaspoon salt, and sauté until the onion is softened and lightly caramelized, about 8 minutes. Add the garlic and sauté for 30 seconds.

2. Add the broth, lentils, tomatoes, spice mixture, black pepper, and the remaining 1/2 teaspoon salt, and bring to a boil over high heat. Reduce heat to medium-low and simmer, uncovered, until the lentils are tender, about 30 minutes. Stir in the spinach and simmer until the spinach is wilted, about 2 minutes. Stir in the yogurt (if using).

3. Ladle into individual bowls, sprinkle with desired amount of the lemon zest, and serve.

{ WITH POULTRY, FISH, OR MEAT }

One serving: Brush a 2 1/2-ounce piece of center-cut, skinned salmon fillet with 1/2 teaspoon extra-virgin olive oil; cut into 4 cubes and insert onto a metal or water-soaked bamboo skewer. Add a smidgen of sea salt and freshly ground black pepper. Grill or pan-grill the kebab over medium-high heat until just cooked through, about 5 minutes. Serve atop one of the bowls of stew, or add the salmon cubes to the stew when serving.

Full recipe: Brush two 7 1/2-ounce center-cut, skinned salmon fillets with 1 tablespoon extra-virgin olive oil; cut each fillet into 12 cubes and insert 4 cubes onto each of 6 metal or water-soaked bamboo skewers. Sprinkle the kebabs with 1/4 teaspoon sea salt and 1/4 teaspoon freshly ground black pepper. Grill or pan-grill the kebabs over medium-high heat until just cooked through, about 5 minutes. Serve a kebab on each bowl of stew, or add the salmon cubes to the stew when serving.

without
Exchanges/Food Choices: 1 Starch, 1 Vegetable, 1/2 Fat
130 calories, 20 calories from fat, 2.5g total fat, 0g saturated fat, 0g trans fat, 0mg cholesterol, 450mg sodium, 540mg potassium, 22g total carbohydrate, 6g dietary fiber, 5g sugars, 7g protein, 40mg phosphorus

with
Exchanges/Food Choices: 1 Starch, 1 Vegetable, 3 Lean Meat, 1 Fat
270 calories, 90 calories from fat, 10g total fat, 1.5g saturated fat, 0g trans fat, 45mg cholesterol, 580mg sodium, 940mg potassium, 23g total carbohydrate, 6g dietary fiber, 5g sugars, 23g protein, 200mg phosphorus

South Asian Spice Trio

Makes 5 servings: 1 teaspoon each

2 teaspoons ground cumin*   1 teaspoon ground turmeric
2 teaspoons ground coriander*

Stir together the cumin, coriander, and turmeric. Store in a labeled jar. Makes 5 teaspoons. Use in Garlic Spinach Dal Stew and other recipes of choice.

*Hint: Instead of buying ground spices, toast whole coriander and cumin seeds and then grind in a coffee grinder or peppermill for a warmer, earthier flavor.

Exchanges/Food Choices: Free Food
5 calories, 2 calories from fat, 0g total fat, 0g saturated fat, 0g trans fat, 0mg cholesterol, 0mg sodium, 20mg potassium, 1g total carbohydrate, 0g dietary fiber, 0g sugars, 0g protein, 5mg phosphorus

California Cannellini Chili

Makes 8 servings: 1 cup chili

1 1/2 teaspoons canola or unrefined peanut oil

1 large red onion, finely diced

1 large green bell pepper, finely diced

1 tablespoon white balsamic or white wine vinegar

3/4 teaspoon sea salt, divided

2 large garlic cloves, minced

1 (14.5-ounce) can crushed roasted tomatoes (1 3/4 cups)

3 cups low-sodium vegetable broth

1/3 cup freshly squeezed orange juice

1 tablespoon + 1 teaspoon chili powder, or to taste

1/2 teaspoon ground cinnamon, or to taste

1/2 teaspoon freshly ground black pepper, or to taste

2 (15-ounce) cans no-salt-added cannellini or other white beans, drained (3 cups)

1/3 cup finely shredded Monterey Jack cheese or vegan cheese alternative

1/2 Hass avocado, peeled, pitted, and finely diced

2 tablespoons roughly chopped fresh cilantro

Chili is usually considered guy-friendly fare, but I wanted to give it a makeover to make it gal-friendly, too. Here's the result! The use of white beans, orange juice, cinnamon, and a topping of avocado is what makes this chili special for all tastes. Want to make it still more special? As an ode to San Francisco, enjoy with whole-grain sourdough bread rolls if you have room for the carbs.

1. Heat the oil in a stockpot over medium-high heat. Add the onion, bell pepper, vinegar, and 1/4 teaspoon salt, and sauté until the onion is lightly caramelized, about 8 minutes. Add the garlic and sauté for 1 minute.

2. Stir in the tomatoes, broth, orange juice, chili powder, cinnamon, black pepper, and the remaining 1/2 teaspoon salt, and bring to a boil over high heat. Reduce heat to medium-low, stir in the beans, and simmer, uncovered, until desired consistency, about 15 minutes. Adjust seasoning.

3. Ladle the chili into individual bowls. Sprinkle with the cheese, avocado, and cilantro, and serve.

{ WITH POULTRY, FISH, OR MEAT }

One serving: Heat 1/2 teaspoon canola oil in a small, nonstick skillet over medium-high heat. Add 2 ounces ground chicken breast and sauté until crumbled and well done, about 2 minutes. Season with a smidgen each of sea salt, freshly ground black pepper, and ground cinnamon. Stir into one of the chili bowls before sprinkling with the cheese.

Full recipe: Heat 1 tablespoon + 1 teaspoon canola oil in a large, nonstick skillet over medium-high heat. Add 1 pound ground chicken breast and sauté until crumbled and well done, about 3 minutes. Season with 1/4 teaspoon each sea salt, freshly ground black pepper, and ground cinnamon. Stir into the chili along with the beans in step 2.

without

Exchanges/Food Choices: 1 Starch, 1 Vegetable, 1 Lean Meat, 1 Fat
170 calories, 40 calories from fat, 4.5g total fat, 1g saturated fat, 0g trans fat, 5mg cholesterol, 480mg sodium, 370mg potassium, 25g total carbohydrate, 7g dietary fiber, 6g sugars, 8g protein, 120mg phosphorus

with

Exchanges/Food Choices: 1 Starch, 1 Vegetable, 2 Lean Meat, 1 Fat
170 calories, 40 calories from fat, 4.5g total fat, 1g saturated fat, 0g trans fat, 5mg cholesterol, 480mg sodium, 370mg potassium, 25g total carbohydrate, 7g dietary fiber, 6g sugars, 8g protein, 120mg phosphorus

Spicy Gameday Chili

Makes 8 servings: 1 cup each

2 teaspoons grapeseed or canola oil

3 cups finely chopped purple or white cauliflower florets

1 large yellow onion, finely diced

2 teaspoons apple cider vinegar

3/4 teaspoon sea salt, divided

1 small jalapeño pepper, with some seeds, minced

2 large garlic cloves, minced

1 (32-fluid ounce) carton low-sodium vegetable broth

1 (14.5-ounce) can crushed roasted tomatoes (1 3/4 cups)

1 1/2 tablespoons chili powder, or to taste

2 teaspoons unsweetened cocoa powder

1/2 teaspoon ground pumpkin pie spice or cinnamon, or to taste

1 (15-ounce) can no-salt-added red kidney or black beans, drained (1 1/2 cups)

2 tablespoons roughly chopped fresh flat-leaf parsley or minced fresh chives

Here's a nicely spiced chili that goes beyond any ordinary chili. The cocoa powder and pumpkin pie spice create flavor intrigue. The cauliflower provides extra body in a healthy way. If you can find purple cauliflower, pick it up. It contains anthocyanins, which have shown promise in reducing the risk of diabetes, heart disease, cancer, and more. This cup of comfort is perfect as is. Or serve it on football gameday along with a buffet of fun toppings. Enjoy it ladled over whole-grain spaghetti as Cincinnati-style chili, too.

1. Heat the oil in a stockpot over medium-high heat. Add the cauliflower, onion, vinegar, and 1/4 teaspoon salt, and sauté until the onion begins to caramelize, about 8 minutes. Add the jalapeño and garlic, and sauté until fragrant, about 30 seconds.

2. Stir in the broth, tomatoes, chili powder, cocoa powder, pumpkin pie spice, and the remaining 1/2 teaspoon salt, and bring to a boil over high heat. Reduce heat to medium-low, stir in the beans, and simmer, uncovered, until desired consistency, about 15 minutes. Adjust seasoning.

3. Ladle the chili into individual bowls, sprinkle with the parsley, and serve.

{ WITH POULTRY, FISH, OR MEAT }

One serving: Heat about 1/2 teaspoon grapeseed or canola oil in a small, nonstick skillet over medium-high heat. Add 1 1/2 ounces lean, ground, grass-fed beef sirloin and sauté until crumbled and well done, about 1 1/2 minutes. Season with a smidgen each of pumpkin pie spice, chili powder, and freshly ground black pepper. Stir into one of the chili bowls before sprinkling with the parsley.

Full recipe: Heat 1 tablespoon grapeseed or canola oil in a large, nonstick skillet over medium-high heat. Add 12 ounces lean, ground, grass-fed beef sirloin and sauté until crumbled and well done, about 2 minutes. Season with 1/4 teaspoon each pumpkin pie spice, chili powder, and freshly ground black pepper. Stir into the chili along with the beans in step 2.

without
Exchanges/Food Choices: 1 Starch, 1/2 Vegetable, 1/2 Fat
100 calories, 20 calories from fat, 2g total fat, 0g saturated fat, 0g trans fat, 0mg cholesterol, 400mg sodium, 370mg potassium, 17g total carbohydrate, 5g dietary fiber, 5g sugars, 5g protein, 80mg phosphorus

with
Exchanges/Food Choices: 1 Starch, 1 Vegetable, 2 Lean Meat
170 calories, 50 calories from fat, 6g total fat, 1.5g saturated fat, 0g trans fat, 25mg cholesterol, 420mg sodium, 480mg potassium, 17g total carbohydrate, 5g dietary fiber, 5g sugars, 13g protein, 140mg phosphorus

Chilled Persian Cucumber Soup with Chives

Makes 4 servings: 1 cup each

2 Persian or 1 English cucumber, unpeeled and coarsely grated

1 1/4 cups plain fat-free Greek yogurt

2 tablespoons + 1 teaspoon minced fresh chives

1 tablespoon finely chopped fresh mint leaves

1 shallot, minced

1 large garlic clove, minced

1 1/2 tablespoons white balsamic or champagne vinegar

3/4 teaspoon freshly ground black pepper, or to taste

1/2 teaspoon sea salt, or to taste

2/3 cup unsweetened green tea or jasmine green tea (made with 1 tea bag), chilled

without
Exchanges/Food Choices: 1/2 Carbohydrate, 1 Vegetable
70 calories, 5 calories from fat, 0g total fat, 0g saturated fat, 0g trans fat, 5mg cholesterol, 320mg sodium, 290mg potassium, 9g total carbohydrate, 1g dietary fiber, 5g sugars, 8g protein, 130mg phosphorus

with
Exchanges/Food Choices: 1/2 Carbohydrate, 1 Vegetable, 2 Lean Meat
140 calories, 40 calories from fat, 4.5g total fat, 1g saturated fat, 0g trans fat, 20mg cholesterol, 410mg sodium, 360mg potassium, 14g total carbohydrate, 1g dietary fiber, 5g sugars, 13g protein, 200mg phosphorus

If you enjoy tzatziki, this full-flavored recipe is like a tangy, cool soup version of it. The grated cucumber along with the unique inclusion of tea makes it refreshing and almost spa-like. What's more, this soup provides bonus health benefits from the green tea, which studies find may help reduce the risk of developing type 2 diabetes.

1. Stir together the cucumber, yogurt, 2 tablespoons chives, the mint, shallot, garlic, vinegar, pepper, salt, and tea in a medium bowl. Adjust seasoning. Chill until ready to serve.

2. Divide the soup among individual small soup cups or bowls. Serve topped with the remaining 1 teaspoon chives.

WITH POULTRY, FISH, OR MEAT

One serving: Place 3 packaged or homemade fully cooked whole-grain chicken nuggets, like the chicken version of Oven-Fried Nuggets (skip the marinara; page 47), onto a bamboo skewer or 3 small skewers; enjoy with the soup fondue-style.

Full recipe: Divide 12 packaged or homemade fully cooked whole-grain chicken nuggets, like the chicken version of Oven-Fried Nuggets (skip the marinara; page 47), among 4 bamboo skewers or 12 small skewers; enjoy with the soup fondue-style.

CHAPTER 5

sandwiches, wraps, and burgers

Roasted Vegetable Wrap

Makes 2 servings: 1 wrap each

2 large portabella mushroom caps, sliced

2 medium bell peppers, preferably 1 red and 1 orange or yellow, sliced

2 large garlic cloves, minced

2 teaspoons canola or extra-virgin olive oil

3/4 teaspoon finely chopped fresh rosemary

1/4 teaspoon freshly ground black pepper, or to taste

1/8 teaspoon sea salt, or to taste

3 tablespoons hummus of choice (page 59)

1 teaspoon aged balsamic vinegar

2 (8-inch) whole-wheat flour tortillas

1 scallion, green and white parts, minced

When you've got lots of sandwich filling, often the best way to enjoy it is all wrapped up. This wrap is definitely a stuffed one! The rosemary-roasted mushrooms and bell peppers provide a sweet-savory pairing that'll win over your appetite. The spread—which is a zingy mixture of hummus and balsamic vinegar—provides creaminess, tanginess, and full-bodied goodness. For easier eating after making the wraps, roll each up in unbleached parchment paper and peel down the paper as you bite into this bodacious delight.

1. Preheat the oven to 450°F. In a large bowl, toss together the mushrooms, bell peppers, garlic, oil, rosemary, black pepper, and salt. Arrange in a single layer on a large unbleached parchment paper–lined baking sheet. Roast until the vegetables are fully cooked, about 20 minutes. (Note: Prepare in advance and chill, if desired.)

2. Mix together the hummus and balsamic vinegar in a small bowl until well combined. Spread the entire surface of each tortilla with the hummus mixture. Sprinkle each with the scallion and the roasted vegetables (warm or cool). Tightly roll up without tucking in sides.

3. Slice in half on the diagonal, and serve at room temperature.

{ WITH POULTRY, FISH, OR MEAT }

One serving: Use 1 1/2 portabella mushroom caps instead of 2 in main recipe. Toss four 1/2-ounce, long, thin strips of boneless, skinless chicken breast with 1/2 teaspoon canola or extra-virgin olive oil and a pinch each of freshly ground black pepper and finely chopped fresh rosemary. Roast in a small pan, lined with unbleached parchment paper, on a rack below the vegetables until done, about 10 minutes. Add to one of the wraps along with the vegetables in step 2.

Full recipe: Use 1 portabella mushroom cap instead of 2 in main recipe. Toss eight 1/2-ounce, long, thin strips of boneless, skinless chicken breast with 1 teaspoon canola or extra-virgin olive oil and 1/8 teaspoon each freshly ground black pepper and finely chopped fresh rosemary. Roast in a small pan, lined with unbleached parchment paper, on a rack below the vegetables until done, about 10 minutes. Add to the wraps along with the vegetables in step 2.

without
Exchanges/Food Choices: 2 Starch, 1 Vegetable, 1 Lean Meat, 1 Fat
260 calories, 90 calories from fat, 10g total fat, 2g saturated fat, 0g trans fat, 0mg cholesterol, 570mg sodium, 710mg potassium, 36g total carbohydrate, 8g dietary fiber, 9g sugars, 9g protein, 250mg phosphorus

with
Exchanges/Food Choices: 2 Starch, 2 Vegetable, 2 Lean Meat, 2 Fat
340 calories, 120 calories from fat, 14g total fat, 2.5g saturated fat, 0g trans fat, 30mg cholesterol, 590mg sodium, 655mg potassium, 34g total carbohydrate, 8g dietary fiber, 7g sugars, 20g protein, 280mg phosphorus

Chimichurri Hummus and Cauliflower Wrap

Makes 2 servings: 1 wrap each

1/2 cup hummus of choice (page 59)

2 tablespoons finely chopped fresh flat-leaf parsley

1 teaspoon finely chopped fresh oregano leaves

1 large garlic clove, minced

2 teaspoons extra-virgin olive oil, divided

1/2 teaspoon red wine vinegar

1/8 teaspoon freshly ground black pepper, or to taste

1/8 teaspoon dried hot pepper flakes, or to taste

2 cups small bite-size cauliflower florets

1/8 teaspoon sea salt, or to taste

2 (8-inch) whole-grain or flax tortillas or soft flatbreads of choice

1/4 cup very thinly sliced red onion

2/3 cup cherry tomatoes, quartered

Caramelized cauliflower is one of the key ingredients in this delightful entrée wrap. The other is hummus, which goes beyond being an ordinary spread. It's not just plain, but turned into a full-flavored chimichurri-inspired hummus by way of parsley, oregano, garlic, vinegar, and hot pepper flakes. Paired with the veggies, it makes this one extraordinary wrap.

1. Stir together the hummus, parsley, oregano, garlic, 1 teaspoon oil, the vinegar, black pepper, and hot pepper flakes until well combined. Adjust seasoning. Set aside.

2. Heat the remaining 1 teaspoon oil in a large, non-stick skillet over medium-high heat. Add the cauliflower and salt, cover, and cook while shaking the pan or stirring occasionally until cooked through and well caramelized, about 7 minutes.

3. Spread the hummus over the entire surface of the tortillas. Sprinkle with the onion, cauliflower (preferably while warm), and tomatoes. Wrap, and serve.

{ WITH POULTRY, FISH, OR MEAT }

One serving: Grill a 2-ounce, thin, lean, grass-fed beef top round "pepper steak" strip over direct medium-high heat until medium-rare, about 1 minute per side. Let stand at least 5 minutes. Slice into thin, matchstick-size pieces. Sprinkle with a pinch of freshly ground black pepper. Add to one of the wraps after spreading with the hummus in step 3.

Full recipe: Grill two 2-ounce, thin, lean, grass-fed beef top round "pepper steak" strips over direct medium-high heat until medium-rare, about 1 minute per side. Let stand at least 5 minutes. Slice into thin, matchstick-size pieces. Sprinkle with 1/8 teaspoon freshly ground black pepper. Add to the wraps after spreading with the hummus in step 3.

without

Exchanges/Food Choices: 2 Starch, 1 1/2 Vegetable, 2 Medium-Fat Meat
320 calories, 120 calories from fat, 14g total fat, 1.5g saturated fat, 0g trans fat, 0mg cholesterol, 490mg sodium, 520mg potassium, 39g total carbohydrate, 9g dietary fiber, 5g sugars, 11g protein, 250mg phosphorus

with

Exchanges/Food Choices: 2 Starch, 1 1/2 Vegetable, 3 Medium-Fat Meat, 1 Fat
390 calories, 140 calories from fat, 16g total fat, 2g saturated fat, 0g trans fat, 30mg cholesterol, 520mg sodium, 710mg potassium, 39g total carbohydrate, 9g dietary fiber, 5g sugars, 24g protein, 370mg phosphorus

Maitake Gyro

Makes 4 servings: 1 gyro (1/2 stuffed pita) each

1/3 cup tahini

1/4 cup unsweetened green tea or water, chilled

Juice of 1/2 small lemon (1 tablespoon), divided

1 small garlic clove, minced

1 teaspoon minced fresh mint

1/4 teaspoon sea salt, divided

1 teaspoon extra-virgin olive oil

12 ounces fresh maitake mushrooms, separated, or sliced mushroom mixture

1 teaspoon finely chopped fresh oregano leaves

1 teaspoon freshly ground black pepper, or to taste

2 large whole-grain pitas, halved, warm

1 cup very thinly sliced unpeeled English cucumber

1 medium vine-ripened tomato, thinly sliced

1/3 cup very thinly sliced red onion

One of my go-to late-night bites in college was the gyro. Since I'm no longer fond of processed gyro meat, I've created many meat-free versions. This is my newest vegan creation. It's inspired by the gyro and is meant to have its own distinct and inviting taste, not imitate the taste. The sautéed maitake mushrooms are so savory and inviting. The other unique addition is green tea. It makes the tahini sauce saucy. Plus, when green tea is paired with starchy food, like pita bread, it may help prevent blood glucose spikes!

1. Stir together with a fork the tahini, tea, 1/2 tablespoon lemon juice, the garlic, mint, and 1/8 teaspoon salt in a liquid measuring cup or small bowl until smooth. Adjust seasoning. Set aside.

2. Heat the oil in a large, nonstick skillet over medium-high heat. Add the mushrooms, oregano, pepper, and the remaining 1/8 teaspoon salt, and sauté until the mushrooms are fully softened and browned, about 6 minutes. Stir in the remaining 1/2 tablespoon lemon juice. Adjust seasoning.

3. Spoon half of the tahini sauce into the pita halves. Stuff with the cucumber, mushrooms, tomato, and onion. Serve with the remaining sauce on the side.

{ WITH POULTRY, FISH, OR MEAT }

One serving: Spritz a small, nonstick skillet with cooking spray and place over medium-high heat. Add a 1-ounce thinly sliced piece of grass-fed lamb loin and sauté until done, about 1 minute. Add a smidgen each of sea salt and black pepper. Slice into bite-size pieces, if desired. Add to one of the pitas along with the mushrooms.

Full recipe: In step 2, after sautéing the mushrooms for about 4 minutes, add 4 ounces very thinly sliced, bite-size pieces of grass-fed lamb loin and sauté until the mushrooms and lamb are done. Add an extra 1/8 teaspoon each sea salt and black pepper.

without
Exchanges/Food Choices: 1 Starch, 1 1/2 Vegetable, 1 Lean Meat, 2 Fat
260 calories, 120 calories from fat, 13g total fat, 2g saturated fat, 0g trans fat, 0mg cholesterol, 310mg sodium, 450mg potassium, 32g total carbohydrate, 7g dietary fiber, 4g sugars, 9g protein, 280mg phosphorus

with
Exchanges/Food Choices: 2 Starch, 1 Vegetable, 2 Lean Meat, 2 Fat
290 calories, 130 calories from fat, 14g total fat, 2.5g saturated fat, 0g trans fat, 15mg cholesterol, 400mg sodium, 510mg potassium, 32g total carbohydrate, 7g dietary fiber, 4g sugars, 13g protein, 320mg phosphorus

Fresh Veggie Club Sandwich

Makes 2 servings: 1 sandwich each

3 tablespoons hummus of choice (page 59)

1/2 teaspoon lemon zest

1/2 teaspoon freshly ground black pepper, or to taste

4 slices hearty whole-grain bread, fresh or toasted

1/4 cup coarsely grated carrot

1/2 Hass avocado, pitted, peeled, and sliced

Pinch sea salt (optional)

1 Kirby cucumber or 5-ounce portion English cucumber, unpeeled, very thinly sliced into "coins" (about 1 cup sliced)

4 thin slices red onion, separated

1 vine-ripened plum tomato, sliced

2 ounces ready-to-eat smoked tofu, very thinly sliced

1 cup packed fresh baby kale, watercress, or mâche (1 ounce)

One of the best things about veggies for people watching their weight is that they provide volume. They can be piled into a sandwich to make it extra satisfying for fewer calories, as you'll discover in this pleasingly stuffed club. If you want to eat this sandwich neatly, wrap it up (try unbleached parchment paper and foil) and peel down the wrapping as you eat it. Otherwise, indulge in all of its glorious freshness, creaminess, and crispness.

1. Stir together the hummus, lemon zest, and pepper in a small bowl. Spread onto one side of all 4 bread slices.

2. Onto 2 bread slices sprinkle half of the carrot. Add the avocado and sprinkle with the salt (if using). Layer on the cucumber, onion, tomato, tofu, kale, and the remaining half of the carrot.

3. Firmly place remaining bread slices on top, cut diagonally in half, secure each half with a toothpick, and serve.

One serving: In one of the sandwiches, use 1 1/2 ounces smoked turkey breast in place of 1 ounce smoked tofu.

Full recipe: Use 3 ounces smoked turkey breast in place of the smoked tofu.

without
Exchanges/Food Choices: 2 Starch, 1 Vegetable, 2 Lean Meat, 1 Fat
310 calories, 100 calories from fat, 12g total fat, 2g saturated fat, 0g trans fat, 0mg cholesterol, 380mg sodium, 720mg potassium, 40g total carbohydrate, 11g dietary fiber, 8g sugars, 16g protein, 280mg phosphorus

with
Exchanges/Food Choices: 2 Starch, 2 Vegetable, 2 Lean Meat, 1 Fat
320 calories, 90 calories from fat, 10g total fat, 1.5g saturated fat, 0g trans fat, 20mg cholesterol, 570mg sodium, 750mg potassium, 38g total carbohydrate, 10g dietary fiber, 7g sugars, 22g protein, 290mg phosphorus

Keep a Cut Avocado Fresh

Only need part of an avocado for a recipe? Once cut open, it will begin to brown. To help prevent discoloration, sprinkle or rub the cut portion with fresh lemon or lime juice, store in an airtight container or wrap well in plastic wrap, and chill in the refrigerator. The natural acids from the citrus juice can keep the cut surface of the avocado green for up to 3 days. But if it does discolor, all you need to do is slice off the top layer.

Po' Boy-Inspired Sandwich

Makes 4 servings: 1 sandwich each

1/4 cup plain fat-free Greek yogurt

1 tablespoon mayonnaise

1 teaspoon horseradish mustard or Creole mustard

1 teaspoon fresh lemon juice

2 scallions, green and white parts, minced

1/2 teaspoon freshly ground black pepper

1/8 teaspoon ground cayenne pepper, or to taste

4 (4-inch) portions whole-grain French baguettes, split

2 cups packed wild baby arugula or mixed baby greens (2 ounces)

12 Oven-Fried Nuggets (skip the marinara; page 46) or 8 prepared meatless crispy "chicken" tenders

1 Hass avocado, pitted, peeled, and sliced

1 teaspoon lemon zest

A po' boy is a popular Louisianan sub sandwich which consists of a baguette that's often stuffed with fried shrimp or oysters. This recipe is loosely inspired by it and is popular in my Brooklyn kitchen. Instead of a doughy baguette, you'll be forming baguette shells, so you'll have just enough bread to hold the filling, which is the highlight here. There's a zippy sauce, oven-fried nuggets, peppery greens, and creamy avocado. All at once, it's a mouthful of joy.

1. Stir together the yogurt, mayonnaise, mustard, lemon juice, scallions, black pepper, and cayenne in a small bowl until well combined.

2. Pinch out the doughy bread from inside the baguettes to form about 1 1/2-ounce baguettes, which will resemble bread shells. Reserve the doughy part for other use, such as making bread-crumbs or croutons.

3. Spread the yogurt sauce into the baguette shells. Layer the bottom portions with the arugula, nuggets, and avocado, and sprinkle with the lemon zest. Place on the baguette tops, and serve.

{ WITH POULTRY, FISH, OR MEAT }

One serving: Into one of the baguettes, swap 3 Oven-Fried Nuggets with 3 prepared, packaged, or homemade fully cooked whole-grain chicken nuggets, like the chicken version of Oven-Fried Nuggets (skip the marinara; page 47).

Full recipe: Into each of the baguettes, swap the Oven-Fried Nuggets with packaged or homemade fully cooked whole-grain chicken nuggets, like the chicken version of Oven-Fried Nuggets (skip the marinara; page 47). (You'll need 12 chicken nuggets total.)

without
Exchanges/Food Choices: 2 Starch, 2 Vegetable, 2 Lean Meat
310 calories, 90 calories from fat, 10g total fat, 1.5g saturated fat, 0g trans fat, 5mg cholesterol, 560mg sodium, 650mg potassium, 42g total carbohydrate, 9g dietary fiber, 6g sugars, 14g protein, 230mg phosphorus

with
Exchanges/Food Choices: 2 Starch, 2 Vegetable, 3 Lean Meat
340 calories, 100 calories from fat, 11g total fat, 2g saturated fat, 0g trans fat, 25mg cholesterol, 580mg sodium, 470mg potassium, 39g total carbohydrate, 8g dietary fiber, 5g sugars, 21g protein, 220mg phosphorus

Italian-Style Submarines

Makes 8 servings: 1 sandwich each

1/2 cup Italian Sandwich Spread (page 147)

8 whole-wheat frankfurter buns, split, lightly toasted

1 ounce drained, thinly sliced pepperoncini or hot Italian peppers

2 cups packed fresh field greens or frisée (2 ounces)

6 ounces very thinly sliced ready-to-eat smoked or Italian baked tofu

3 ounces thinly sliced provolone cheese

1 1/2 cups packed shredded radicchio (2 ounces)

Hosting a party? Here's a fun recipe designed for a casual gathering of kids, adults, or both. Perfectly portioned hot dog buns are used for these personal-sized sub sandwiches. But instead of mustard and hot dogs, you'll be smearing a tangy herb spread into these cute veggie-friendly submarines. You'll be amazed at how much flavor is packed into each bite.

1. Smear the sandwich spread into the buns.

2. Layer onto the bottom portion of the buns the pepperoncini, field greens, tofu, cheese, and radicchio. Firmly place on the bun tops, and serve.

{ WITH POULTRY, FISH, OR MEAT }

One serving: Add 3/4 ounce extra-thinly sliced rosemary ham, prosciutto, or American country ham onto one of the buns instead of the smoked tofu. (You'll only need 5 1/4 ounces smoked tofu for the rest of the submarines.)

Full recipe: Layer 3/4 ounce extra-thinly sliced rosemary ham, prosciutto, or American country ham onto each of the buns instead of the smoked tofu. (You'll need 6 ounces ham total.)

Italian Sandwich Spread

Makes 8 servings: 1 tablespoon each

3 tablespoons hummus
of choice

3 tablespoons plain fat-free
Greek yogurt

2 large garlic cloves, minced

3 tablespoons chopped fresh
basil

1 tablespoon chopped fresh
oregano leaves

2 teaspoons aged balsamic
vinegar

1/2 teaspoon freshly ground
black pepper, or to taste

Stir together the hummus, yogurt, garlic, basil, oregano, vinegar, and black pepper in a small bowl. Makes 1/2 cup. Use as a condiment for Italian-Style Submarines or sandwich of choice.

Exchanges/Food Choices: Free Food
15 calories, 5 calories from fat, 0.5g total fat, 0g saturated fat, 0g trans fat, 0mg cholesterol, 25mg sodium, 30mg potassium, 2g total carbohydrate, 0g dietary fiber, 0g sugars, 1g protein, 20mg phosphorus

without
Exchanges/Food Choices: 2 Starch, 1 Vegetable, 1 Medium-Fat Meat
200 calories, 60 calories from fat, 7g total fat, 2.5g saturated fat, 0g trans fat, 10mg cholesterol, 470mg sodium, 250mg potassium, 26g total carbohydrate, 4g dietary fiber, 5g sugars, 11g protein, 220mg phosphorus

with
Exchanges/Food Choices: 1 1/2 Starch, 2 Lean Meat
190 calories, 50 calories from fat, 6g total fat, 2.5g saturated fat, 0g trans fat, 15mg cholesterol, 590mg sodium, 270mg potassium, 25g total carbohydrate, 4g dietary fiber, 5g sugars, 12g protein, 220mg phosphorus

Mozzarella, Arugula, and Plum Ciabatta

Makes 4 servings: 1 sandwich each

1 (8-ounce) whole-grain ciabatta or whole-grain baguette, split

1 tablespoon + 1 teaspoon aged balsamic vinegar

2 teaspoons extra-virgin olive oil

2 cups packed fresh baby arugula, divided (2 ounces)

1/4 cup very thinly sliced red onion

2 medium fresh purple plums or yellow peaches, halved, seeded, and thinly sliced

1/2 teaspoon freshly ground black pepper, or to taste

2 ounces sliced part-skim mozzarella cheese

without

Exchanges/Food Choices: 1 1/2 Starch, 1 Medium-Fat Meat

200 calories, 60 calories from fat, 6g total fat, 2g saturated fat, 0g trans fat, 10mg cholesterol, 260mg sodium, 240mg potassium, 26g total carbohydrate, 4g dietary fiber, 8g sugars, 10g protein, 170mg phosphorus

with

Exchanges/Food Choices: 2 Starch, 2 Lean Meat

220 calories, 60 calories from fat, 7g total fat, 2.5g saturated fat, 0g trans fat, 15mg cholesterol, 510mg sodium, 290mg potassium, 26g total carbohydrate, 4g dietary fiber, 8g sugars, 12g protein, 200mg phosphorus

Plums are what make this stuffed ciabatta sandwich so special. The fruity sweetness is balanced by the pepperiness of the greens, sharpness of the onion, tanginess of the balsamic vinegar, and saltiness of the cheese. It's okay to use plums or peaches that aren't fully ripened if you prefer a not-so-sweet sandwich filling. You can also make this memorable recipe with one large pear or apple instead of the two plums or peaches for a seasonal change of taste.

1. Pinch out 2 ounces doughy bread from inside the ciabatta, forming a 6-ounce loaf. Reserve the doughy part for other use, such as making croutons.

2. Drizzle the cut surfaces of the ciabatta with the vinegar and oil.

3. Layer onto the bottom portion of the ciabatta 1 cup arugula. Then top with the onion and plums. Sprinkle with the pepper. Top with the mozzarella and the remaining 1 cup arugula.

4. Firmly add the ciabatta top, slice into 4 sandwiches, skewer with bamboo or reusable picks, if desired, and serve.

WITH POULTRY, FISH, OR MEAT

One serving: After cutting into 4 sandwiches, add 1/3 ounce extra-thinly sliced prosciutto or American country ham into one of the sandwiches.

Full recipe: Layer 1 1/3 ounces extra-thinly sliced prosciutto or American country ham into the whole sandwich between the cheese and arugula at the end of step 3 (1/3 ounce prosciutto in each).

Roquefort, Mizuna, and Pear Toastie

Makes 4 servings: 1 sandwich each

Looking to entice all of your senses at once? Look no further. This toastie recipe will awaken your taste buds and so much more with its crisp pear, pungent cheese, bright greens, and perfect touch of aromatic rosemary. Simple yet sensational!

1. Toast the bread slices. Immediately top all toast slices with the cheese.

2. Toss the mizuna with the vinegar in a medium bowl.

3. Top 4 of the slices with the rosemary, pear, and dressed mizuna. Place the other toast slices onto the mizuna, cheese side down; firmly press to form a sandwich, and serve.

WITH POULTRY, FISH, OR MEAT

One serving: Top one of the toasted bread slices with 1 ounce thinly sliced smoked peppercorn turkey, cold applewood smoked magret de canard (smoked duck breast), or shaved smoked pork loin immediately following the cheese.

Full recipe: Top 4 of the toasted bread slices with 1 ounce thinly sliced smoked peppercorn turkey, cold applewood-smoked magret de canard (smoked duck breast), or shaved smoked pork loin immediately following the cheese. (You'll need 4 ounces turkey, duck, or pork total.)

8 (1-ounce) slices sprouted or whole-grain sourdough bread

1 1/2 ounces crumbled or very thinly sliced Roquefort or gorgonzola cheese, at room temperature

2 cups packed mizuna or baby arugula (2 ounces)

1 teaspoon aged balsamic vinegar

3/4 teaspoon finely chopped fresh rosemary

1 Bosc or other pear, cored, very thinly sliced, at room temperature

without
Exchanges/Food Choices: 2 Starch,
1 Medium-Fat Meat
200 calories, 40 calories from fat, 4.5g total fat,
2g saturated fat, 0g trans fat, 10mg cholesterol,
320mg sodium, 240mg potassium, 33g total
carbohydrate, 7g dietary fiber, 5g sugars,
9g protein, 180mg phosphorus

with
Exchanges/Food Choices: 2 Starch, 1 Lean Meat,
1/2 Fat
230 calories, 40 calories from fat, 4.5g total fat,
2g saturated fat, 0g trans fat, 20mg cholesterol,
490mg sodium, 320mg potassium, 33g total
carbohydrate, 7g dietary fiber, 5g sugars,
16g protein, 220mg phosphorus

Spinach-Artichoke Panini

Makes 2 servings: 1 sandwich each

4 ounces frozen artichoke hearts

3 cups packed fresh baby spinach (3 ounces)

1/2 teaspoon lemon zest

Pinch sea salt (optional)

3 tablespoons shredded pepper jack cheese

2 teaspoons grated Pecorino Romano or Parmigiano-Reggiano cheese

4 (1-ounce) slices whole-grain sourdough bread

2 thin slices medium red onion, separated

Cooking spray

1 large garlic clove, peeled, halved

Spinach-artichoke dip is a favorite for many. Unfortunately, it's scandalously rich. So I decided to bring its highlights into a scandal-free sandwich that can be indulged in often. The spiciness of the pepper jack and sharpness of the Romano bring extra flavor, the lemon zest creates lovely brightness, and the onion brings a little bite. Brought together into a toasty panini with artichoke hearts and baby spinach, this recipe may become a new favorite.

1. Prepare the artichoke hearts according to package directions. Drain, thinly slice, and set aside.

2. Add the spinach to a large, nonstick skillet over medium heat. Toss until the spinach is fully wilted, about 2 1/2 minutes. Transfer to a bowl, sprinkle with the lemon zest and the salt (if using), and set aside. Drain off excess liquids before using in sandwiches.

3. Sprinkle half of the cheeses among 2 bread slices. Top with the artichoke hearts, onion, spinach, and the remaining cheeses. Add the remaining bread slices to form sandwiches. Lightly spritz both sides of the sandwiches with cooking spray.

4. Preheat a panini grill to medium-high. Place sandwiches onto the grill. Grill until golden brown and the cheese is melted, about 4 minutes. Immediately rub the entire surface of the panini sandwiches with the cut end of the garlic. Slice the paninis in half on the diagonal, if desired, and serve immediately.

{ WITH POULTRY, FISH, OR MEAT }

One serving: Add 1 ounce small chunks of picked-over premium wild claw lump crabmeat or cooked, chilled lobster tail meat into one of the sandwiches in step 3 between the onion and spinach.

Full recipe: Add 2 ounces small chunks of picked-over premium wild claw lump crabmeat or cooked, chilled lobster tail meat into the sandwiches in step 3 between the onion and spinach.

without
Exchanges/Food Choices: 1 1/2 Starch,
2 Vegetable, 1 Medium-Fat Meat
240 calories, 60 calories from fat, 7g total fat,
2.5g saturated fat, 0g trans fat, 15mg cholesterol,
380mg sodium, 570mg potassium, 34g total
carbohydrate, 10g dietary fiber, 5g sugars,
14g protein, 200mg phosphorus

with
Exchanges/Food Choices: 1 1/2 Starch,
2 Vegetable, 2 Lean Meat
260 calories, 60 calories from fat, 7g total fat,
2.5g saturated fat, 0g trans fat, 40mg cholesterol,
500mg sodium, 640mg potassium, 34g total
carbohydrate, 10g dietary fiber, 5g sugars,
19g protein, 260mg phosphorus

Sloppy Sautéed Eggplant and Pepper Sandwich

Makes 4 servings: 1 sandwich each

4 (2-ounce) whole-wheat or other whole-grain sandwich rolls, split

1/4 cup shredded provolone cheese (1 ounce)

2 teaspoons canola or grapeseed oil

1 large (1 1/4-pound) eggplant, unpeeled, cut into 2-inch × 1/2-inch batons

2 large green bell peppers or mixture of green and red bell peppers, thinly sliced

1 medium yellow onion, halved, thinly sliced

3/4 teaspoon freshly ground black pepper, to taste

1 tablespoon white balsamic or white wine vinegar, divided

1/8 teaspoon sea salt, to taste

1/4 cup Spicy Sandwich Spread (page 153)

This is no Sloppy Joe. It's better! The recipe is actually a non-traditional twist on a Philly cheesesteak sandwich, though it's messier and overloaded with delicious veggies instead of beef. The sloppiness of it all makes it seem decadent. To top that off, there's just enough cheese and creamy sauce to add comfort. So get cooking now...this is comfort food worth taking a bite of often!

1. Toast the rolls. Immediately sprinkle with the cheese. Set aside.

2. Heat the oil in a nonstick Dutch oven or large, deep skillet over medium-high heat. Add the eggplant, bell peppers, onion, black pepper, 2 teaspoons vinegar, and the salt. Cover and cook, stirring twice, until the vegetables are slightly softened, about 12 minutes. Uncover and sauté until the vegetables are fully softened, about 5 minutes. Stir in the remaining 1 teaspoon vinegar while scraping up the browned bits in the pan for 1 minute. Adjust seasoning. (Makes about 4 cups.)

3. Smear each bun with the sandwich spread, fill with the vegetables, and enjoy immediately.

One serving: Very thinly slice into strips 2/3 ounce lean, grass-fed roast beef. Top one of the sandwiches with the roast beef strips after topping with the cheese in step 1.

Full recipe: Very thinly slice into strips 2 1/2 ounces lean, grass-fed roast beef. Add to the Dutch oven along with the 1 teaspoon vinegar at the end of step 2.

without
Exchanges/Food Choices: 2 Starch, 2 Vegetable, 1 Lean Meat, 1 Fat
280 calories, 80 calories from fat, 9g total fat, 2g saturated fat, 0g trans fat, 5mg cholesterol, 520mg sodium, 690mg potassium, 45g total carbohydrate, 10g dietary fiber, 13g sugars, 10g protein, 230mg phosphorus

with
Exchanges/Food Choices: 2 Starch, 2 Vegetable, 2 Lean Meat
310 calories, 90 calories from fat, 10g total fat, 2.5g saturated fat, 0g trans fat, 20mg cholesterol, 530mg sodium, 730mg potassium, 45g total carbohydrate, 10g dietary fiber, 13g sugars, 15g protein, 260mg phosphorus

Spicy Sandwich Spread

Makes 4 servings: 1 tablespoon each

2 tablespoons plain fat-free Greek yogurt
1 1/2 teaspoons mayonnaise
1 small Serrano pepper, without seeds, minced

1 large garlic clove, minced
1 teaspoon white balsamic or white wine vinegar
1/8 teaspoon sea salt, to taste

Stir together the yogurt, mayonnaise, Serrano pepper, garlic, vinegar, and salt in a small bowl until well combined. Makes 1/4 cup. Use as the condiment in Sloppy Sautéed Eggplant and Pepper Sandwich and other sandwiches of choice.

Exchanges/Food Choices: Free Food
20 calories, 10 calories from fat, 1.5g total fat, 0g saturated fat, 0g trans fat, 0mg cholesterol, 85mg sodium, 20mg potassium, 1g total carbohydrate, 0g dietary fiber, 0g sugars, 1g protein, 10mg phosphorus

Caprese Avocado "Cheeseburger"

Makes 1 serving: 1 "cheeseburger"

1 whole-grain English muffin or sandwich rounds (thins), split

2 tablespoons shredded part-skim mozzarella cheese

1/4 Hass avocado, sliced

4 large fresh basil leaves

1 large, thin slice of red onion

1/2 cup packed fresh wild or baby arugula

1 teaspoon canola or extra-virgin olive oil, divided

1/2 teaspoon aged balsamic vinegar

1 large portabella mushroom cap

1/8 teaspoon freshly ground black pepper, or to taste

Pinch sea salt or smoked sea salt, or to taste

1 large thick slice beefsteak or heirloom tomato, seeds removed

This is no ordinary cheeseburger. It's piled high with tasty ingredients that are full of texture and color. A smoky portabella mushroom provides amazing meatiness. After you indulge in this savory deluxe "cheeseburger" with Caprese flair from mozzarella, basil, and tomato, you might actually feel healthier. Multiply the recipe by as many as you need. Then, simply open wide!

1. Toast the English muffin halves. Transfer to a plate, cut side up. Immediately sprinkle the cheese on the top half. Arrange the avocado, basil, and onion on the bottom half. Set aside.

2. Toss the arugula with 1/2 teaspoon oil and the balsamic vinegar in a small bowl. Set aside.

3. Rub or brush the rounded side of the mushroom cap with the remaining 1/2 teaspoon oil, then sprinkle the gill side with the pepper and salt. Heat a nonstick skillet over medium-high heat. Cook the mushroom cap, gill side up, covered, for 3 minutes. Reduce to medium heat and cook the mushroom cap gill side down, covered, until fully cooked, about 3 minutes more. Place gill side up on the bottom muffin half.

4. Top with the tomato and dressed arugula. Add the muffin top, and serve immediately.

{ WITH POULTRY, FISH, OR MEAT }

For one serving (full recipe): Combine 2 ounces ground chicken or turkey breast, 1 minced small garlic clove, and an additional 1/4 teaspoon aged balsamic vinegar, and form into a thin patty. Instead of the mushroom cap in step 3, cook the ground chicken patty, uncovered, in the nonstick skillet over medium-high heat in the remaining 1/2 teaspoon oil until well done, about 2 minutes per side. Sprinkle with the pepper and salt.

without
Exchanges/Food Choices: 2 Starch, 1 Vegetable, 1 Medium-Fat Meat, 1 Fat
310 calories, 130 calories from fat, 15g total fat, 3g saturated fat, 0g trans fat, 10mg cholesterol, 490mg sodium, 760mg potassium, 37g total carbohydrate, 9g dietary fiber, 10g sugars, 13g protein, 390mg phosphorus

with
Exchanges/Food Choices: 2 Starch, 1 Vegetable, 2 Lean Meat, 2 Fat
360 calories, 140 calories from fat, 16g total fat, 3g saturated fat, 0g trans fat, 40mg cholesterol, 520mg sodium, 560mg potassium, 35g total carbohydrate, 8g dietary fiber, 8g sugars, 23g protein, 380mg phosphorus

Stewed Green Burrito

Makes 4 servings: 1 burrito each

1 1/2 teaspoons canola or peanut oil

2 medium zucchini, unpeeled, finely chopped

1 small or 1/2 large yellow onion, finely chopped

2 large garlic cloves, minced

3/4 cup medium tomatillo salsa (salsa verde)

1 (15-ounce) can no-salt-added pinto beans, drained (1 1/2 cups)

1/4 teaspoon sea salt, or to taste

1/8 teaspoon ground cumin, or to taste

1 teaspoon finely chopped fresh oregano leaves

3 tablespoons chopped fresh cilantro

4 (8-inch) whole spelt or other whole-grain tortillas, warm

1/3 cup shredded Chihuahua or Monterey Jack cheese

2 cups packed shredded Romaine lettuce (2 ounces)

A burrito can be loaded with calories, but not here. Instead, it's loaded with lots of delicious (and green!) ingredients, including green salsa, zucchini, lettuce, and herbs. In fact, it's so pleasingly stuffed that you shouldn't even try picking this one up. You'll save carb calories by not using an extra-large tortilla.

1. Heat the oil in a large, nonstick skillet over medium-high heat. Add the zucchini and onion, and sauté until the zucchini begins to caramelize and the onion is softened, about 5 minutes. Add the garlic and sauté until fragrant, about 1 minute. Add the salsa, beans, salt, and cumin, and stir for 1 minute to fully combine. Cover, reduce heat to low, and simmer until all the vegetables are fully softened, about 10 minutes.

2. Remove the lid, stir in the oregano, and continue to cook while stirring occasionally until no excess liquid remains, about 5 minutes. Stir in the cilantro. Adjust seasoning.

3. Onto each tortilla, sprinkle the cheese, bean mixture, and lettuce. Roll up tightly without folding in the ends. Secure closed with small bamboo picks, if desired. Enjoy with a fork and knife.

{ WITH POULTRY, FISH, OR MEAT }

One serving: Prepare an indoor or outdoor grill. Grill a 1 1/2-ounce piece of lean pork tenderloin over medium-high heat until cooked medium to medium-well. Let stand for at least 5 minutes before slicing. Cut into extra-thin, matchstick-size strips. Sprinkle into one of the tortillas in step 3 after the cheese.

Full recipe: Prepare an indoor or outdoor grill. Grill a 6-ounce piece of lean pork tenderloin over medium-high heat until cooked medium to medium-well. Let stand for at least 5 minutes before slicing. Cut into extra-thin, matchstick-size strips. Stir into the bean mixture at the beginning of step 2 along with the oregano.

without
Exchanges/Food Choice: 2 Starch, 1 1/2 Vegetable, 1 Medium-Fat Meat, 1/2 Fat
300 calories, 70 calories from fat, 8g total fat, 2g saturated fat, 0g trans fat, 10mg cholesterol, 550mg sodium, 700mg potassium, 43g total carbohydrate, 9g dietary fiber, 6g sugars, 13g protein, 260mg phosphorus

with
Exchanges/Food Choices: 2 1/2 Starch, 1 1/2 Vegetable, 1 Lean Meat, 1 Fat
340 calories, 80 calories from fat, 9g total fat, 2.5g saturated fat, 0g trans fat, 30mg cholesterol, 570mg sodium, 840mg potassium, 43g total carbohydrate, 9g dietary fiber, 6g sugars, 21g protein, 340mg phosphorus

Black Bean and Sweet Potato Quesadilla

Makes 6 serving: 2 wedges each

6 (8-inch) whole-wheat tortillas

Cooking spray

2/3 cup shredded part-skim mozzarella cheese (2 1/2 ounces)

1 1/2 ounces finely crumbled soft goat cheese

1 medium boiled or baked sweet potato with skin, finely diced

1 cup drained canned or cooked black beans

2 scallions, green and white parts, thinly sliced

1/2 small jalapeño pepper, halved lengthwise, seeds removed, extra-thinly sliced crosswise

2 tablespoons finely chopped fresh cilantro

1/2 teaspoon finely chopped fresh oregano leaves (optional)

1/4 teaspoon freshly ground black pepper, or to taste

3/4 cup guacamole of choice (page 159; optional)

Healthful food can be fun, and this quesadilla serves up fun as an entrée. You can also serve it to many folks as a party appetizer, if you prefer. There's just enough cheese to hold the quesadilla together and provide the cheesiness you crave. The sweet potato provides a distinct flavor, and its creaminess creates a more luscious bite. The black beans add heartiness and staying power, and their savory flavor balances the potato's natural sweetness. The flavors will be memorable with or without guacamole.

1. Lay the tortillas onto a clean surface or large cutting board and lightly spray only one side of each with cooking spray. Turn 3 tortillas over and sprinkle the entire surface with half of the mozzarella, half of the goat cheese, the sweet potato, black beans, scallions, jalapeño, cilantro, oregano (if using), black pepper, and the remaining mozzarella and goat cheese. Top with the 3 remaining tortillas, sprayed side up. Firmly press each quesadilla with a spatula to fully compact the ingredients.

2. Cook quesadillas in batches in a large skillet over medium-high heat, until well browned, about 1 1/2–2 minutes per side. Cut each quesadilla into 4 wedges.

3. Serve while warm on individual plates with the guacamole (if using) on the side.

One serving: Finely chop one precooked, shelled, deveined shrimp with tail removed. Sprinkle onto half of one of the tortillas after adding the black beans in step 1.

Full recipe: Finely chop 6 precooked, shelled, deveined shrimp with tail removed. Sprinkle onto the tortillas after adding the black beans in step 1.

without
Exchanges/Food Choices: 2 Starch,
1 Medium-Fat Meat
240 calories, 60 calories from fat, 6g total fat,
2g saturated fat, 0g trans fat, 10mg cholesterol,
320mg sodium, 320mg potassium, 33g total
carbohydrate, 4g dietary fiber, 4g sugars,
11g protein, 220mg phosphorus

with
Exchanges/Food Choices: 2 Starch,
1 Medium-Fat Meat, 1 1/2 Fat
250 calories, 60 calories from fat, 7g total fat,
2.5g saturated fat, 0g trans fat, 20mg cholesterol,
380mg sodium, 330mg potassium, 33g total
carbohydrate, 4g dietary fiber, 4g sugars,
12g protein, 230mg phosphorus

Guacamole

Some recipes suggest using "guacamole of choice" (pages 22, 158, and 186). You can use your favorite store-bought variety, your own recipe, or mine:

Jackie's Hass Avocado Guacamole

Makes 6 servings: 2 tablespoons each

1 Hass avocado, pitted, peeled, and cubed
2 teaspoons fresh lime juice
3 tablespoons finely diced red onion
1 tablespoon chopped fresh cilantro

1/2 small jalapeño pepper, with some seeds, minced
1/4 teaspoon ground coriander
1/4 teaspoon sea salt, or to taste

Stir together all of the ingredients in a medium bowl until combined, and serve. Makes 3/4 cup.

Exchanges/Food Choices: 1 Fat
40 calories, 30 calories from fat, 3.5g total fat, 0g saturated fat, 0g trans fat, 0mg cholesterol, 100mg sodium, 130mg potassium, 3g total carbohydrate, 2g dietary fiber, 0g sugars, 1g protein, 10mg phosphorus

Grilled Truffle, Red Onion, and Rosemary Pizza

Makes 8 servings: 1 piece each

2 1/2 teaspoons white truffle oil or extra-virgin olive oil, divided

1 large red onion, halved, extra-thinly sliced

1 teaspoon minced fresh rosemary

1/4 teaspoon sea salt, or to taste

1/4 teaspoon freshly ground black pepper, or to taste

14 ounces fresh or thawed frozen whole-wheat pizza dough*

3/4 cup shredded part-skim mozzarella cheese (3 ounces)

1/4 cup chopped fresh flat-leaf parsley

I live in Brooklyn, where we have the most amazing pizza. So I'm quite particular when it comes to a good slice. Luckily, I didn't have to compromise when making this recipe. The pizza is extra tasty from the smoky charred crust and the truffle oil. And the caramelized onion topping provides a spectacular savory bite with a hint of sweetness. Better than burgers for your next cookout, this pizza is super tasty prepared indoors anytime using a grill pan, too.

1. Heat 1 1/2 teaspoons oil in a large, nonstick skillet over medium-high heat. Add the onion, rosemary, salt, and pepper, and sauté until the onion is lightly caramelized, about 8 minutes. (Note: If the onion begins to stick to the skillet, cover it to trap in moisture while stirring occasionally.) Transfer to a plate and set aside.

2. Prepare an outdoor or indoor grill or grill pan. Shape the pizza dough into two 9-inch-round thin crusts. Lightly brush or rub both sides of the formed dough with the remaining 1 teaspoon oil.

3. Gently lay the dough onto the grill grates (in batches, if necessary) over direct medium heat and grill for 5 minutes. Then, grill over medium-high heat until the bottom has well-defined, charred grill marks, about 5 minutes more. Flip over, top each crust immediately with the reserved onion and the cheese, cover, and grill over medium-high heat for 2 minutes; rotate to form cross-hatch grill marks on

the crust, and continue to grill, covered, until the crust bottom is browned, dough is cooked through, and cheese is melted, about 2 minutes more.

4. Transfer the pizzas onto a cutting board, adjust seasoning, and slice into 4 pieces each. Sprinkle with the parsley, and serve immediately.

*If you have a pound of dough, bake the remaining 2 ounces into a roll or soft breadstick and enjoy at a later meal. You can also freeze for later use.

{ WITH POULTRY, FISH, OR MEAT }

One serving: Prepare an outdoor or indoor grill or grill pan. Grill a 1-ounce portion of lean, grass-fed, beef tenderloin steak over direct high heat until charred on the outside and rare to medium-rare on the inside, about 1 1/2 minutes per side. Let stand for at least 5 minutes. Thinly slice and sprinkle with a pinch of sea salt and freshly ground black pepper. Arrange onto one-quarter of one of the pizzas during the last 2 minutes of lidded grilling in step 3.

Full recipe: Prepare an outdoor or indoor grill or grill pan. Grill 1 (8-ounce) lean, grass-fed, beef tenderloin steak, about 1 inch thick, over direct high heat until charred on the outside and rare to medium-rare on the inside, about 2 1/2 minutes per side. Let stand for at least 5 minutes. Thinly slice and sprinkle with 1/4 teaspoon each sea salt and freshly ground black pepper. Arrange onto the pizzas during the last 2 minutes of lidded grilling in step 3.

without
Exchanges/Food Choices: 2 Starch,
1 Medium-Fat Meat, 1/2 Fat
230 calories, 70 calories from fat, 8g total fat,
2g saturated fat, 0g trans fat, 5mg cholesterol,
410mg sodium, 210mg potassium, 35g total
carbohydrate, 5g dietary fiber, 3g sugars,
9g protein, 200mg phosphorus

with
Exchanges/Food Choices: 2 Starch,
1 Medium-Fat Meat, 1 Fat
270 calories, 80 calories from fat, 9g total fat,
2.5g saturated fat, 0g trans fat, 25mg cholesterol,
500mg sodium, 280mg potassium, 35g total
carbohydrate, 5g dietary fiber, 3g sugars,
15g protein, 250mg phosphorus

Truffles

Truffles are a prized culinary jewel because of their distinct flavor. They're commonly sourced from France and are famously lavish. They grow in the States, too, notably in Oregon. Fortunately, truffle oil can provide the flavor and aromatic essence. A drizzle is all you need, so you won't need to break the bank! My pick: Oregon Truffle Oil—it's all natural and made with wild Oregon white truffles.

Broccoli Quiche Pocket

Makes 8 servings: 1 pocket each

5 large egg whites or 2/3 cup pasteurized 100% egg whites

5 large organic eggs, divided

2 tablespoons plain fat-free Greek yogurt

1/2 teaspoon + 1/8 teaspoon sea salt, or to taste

1/2 teaspoon freshly ground black pepper, or to taste

2 teaspoons canola or extra-virgin olive oil

1 large red or white onion, finely chopped

3 cups packed chopped broccoli florets and tender stems

1 1/2 cups chopped crimini or white button mushrooms

2 teaspoons white balsamic or champagne vinegar

1/2 cup shredded part-skim mozzarella cheese (2 ounces)

1/4 cup finely chopped fresh flat-leaf parsley

2 teaspoons minced fresh tarragon or basil

3 tablespoons plain unsweetened almond milk or other plant-based milk

8 (8-inch) whole-wheat tortillas

2 teaspoons unsalted butter, melted

Here's a way to satisfy a hankering for quiche. These baked pockets are stuffed with a savory egg, cheese, and broccoli filling, and the "crust" is simply tortillas that become crisp in the oven and laced with the perfect amount of butter for richness. Perhaps the best part is that you can individually freeze each pocket and reheat it in the microwave in just two minutes whenever you like.

1. Whisk together the egg whites, 4 whole eggs, the yogurt, 1/2 teaspoon salt, and the pepper in a medium bowl or large liquid measuring cup. Set aside.

2. Heat the oil in a large, deep, nonstick skillet over medium-high heat. Add the onion, broccoli, mushrooms, vinegar, and the remaining 1/8 teaspoon salt, and sauté until the onion is lightly caramelized and broccoli is just tender, about 12 minutes. Remove the skillet from the heat and immediately add the egg mixture. Scramble until the eggs are still slightly runny, about 45 seconds. (Do not fully cook.) Transfer to a large bowl and stir in the cheese, parsley, and tarragon.

3. Meanwhile, preheat the oven to 425°F. Whisk together the remaining 1 egg and the almond milk in a small bowl or small liquid measuring cup. Brush both sides of each tortilla with the egg–almond milk mixture, using all of the mixture. Alternatively, soak the tortillas in the egg mixture like French toast.

4. Working on a cutting board, place about 1/2 cup scrambled egg–vegetable mixture in the center of each moistened tortilla. Fold the bottom portion of the tortilla over the filling, then fold in the sides, then fold over to form a rectangular shape. Arrange onto an unbleached parchment paper–lined baking pan, seam side down. Flatten slightly by pressing with your hand or the back of a spatula.

5. Bake until the tortillas are golden brown, about 20 minutes. Lightly and immediately brush the pockets with the butter, and serve while warm.

{ WITH POULTRY, FISH, OR MEAT }

One serving: Add 1/2 ounce finely diced smoked turkey breast or lean rosemary ham along with 1/2 cup scrambled egg–vegetable mixture to one of the tortillas in step 4. Sprinkle with 1/8 teaspoon finely chopped fresh tarragon after brushing with the butter in step 5.

Full recipe: Stir 4 ounces finely diced smoked turkey breast or lean rosemary ham into the scrambled egg–vegetable mixture along with the cheese in step 2. Sprinkle with 1 teaspoon finely chopped fresh tarragon after brushing with the butter in step 5.

without
Exchanges/Food Choices: 1 1/2 Starch, 1 Vegetable, 2 Lean Meat
260 calories, 90 calories from fat, 10g total fat, 2.5g saturated fat, 0g trans fat, 125mg cholesterol, 490mg sodium, 340mg potassium, 28g total carbohydrate, 4g dietary fiber, 3g sugars, 14g protein, 230mg phosphorus

with
Exchanges/Food Choices: 1 1/2 Starch, 1 Vegetable, 3 Lean Meat
270 calories, 90 calories from fat, 10g total fat, 2.5g saturated fat, 0g trans fat, 130mg cholesterol, 580mg sodium, 390mg potassium, 28g total carbohydrate, 4g dietary fiber, 3g sugars, 17g protein, 260mg phosphorus

Herb Lovers "Melt"

1 (8-inch) whole-wheat or other whole-grain tortilla

1/4 cup no-salt-added Great Northern or cannellini beans*

2 tablespoons shredded part-skim mozzarella cheese (1/2 ounce)

1 scallion, green and white parts, minced

4 or 5 large fresh basil leaves, thinly sliced

1 teaspoon finely chopped fresh dill or tarragon

Pinch sea salt

Pinch dried hot pepper flakes

1 lemon wedge

without
Exchanges/Food Choices: 2 Starch,
1 Lean Meat
210 calories, 50 calories from fat,
5g total fat, 2.5g saturated fat, 0g trans fat,
10mg cholesterol, 580mg sodium,
260mg potassium, 31g total carbohydrate,
6g dietary fiber, 2g sugars, 11g protein,
200mg phosphorus

with
Exchanges/Food Choices: 2 Starch,
2 Lean Meat
240 calories, 60 calories from fat,
6g total fat, 2.5g saturated fat, 0g trans fat,
20mg cholesterol, 560mg sodium,
320mg potassium, 31g total carbohydrate,
6g dietary fiber, 2g sugars, 15g protein,
230mg phosphorus

When you need a light entrée in a pinch, this fusion-style recipe is the pick, especially if you have fresh herbs growing in your garden or windowsill. It's flavorful, fragrant, and fast. But do slow down to enjoy it—with a fork and knife!

1. Place the tortilla on a microwave-safe plate. Sprinkle the entire surface of the tortilla with the beans, cheese, scallion, basil, dill, salt, and hot pepper flakes. Microwave on high until the cheese is melted and beans are fully heated, about 30 seconds.

2. Fold in half, squirt with the lemon, and serve.

*Note: Put the remaining portion of beans to other use, such as to make a simple bean salad side by tossing them lightly with vinaigrette and basil.

WITH POULTRY, FISH, OR MEAT

For one serving (full recipe): Use only 1 rounded tablespoon cheese and do not add the salt in the main recipe. Spritz a small, nonstick skillet with olive oil cooking spray and place over medium-high heat. Add 1 ounce ground turkey (about 94% lean) and sauté until well crumbled and fully cooked, about 2 minutes. Add 1/8 teaspoon freshly ground black pepper and a pinch of sea salt. Sprinkle onto the tortilla at the end of step 1, before folding.

CHAPTER 6
main dishes

Satay Zucchini Noodles

Makes 1 serving: 3 cups

2 medium zucchini or yellow summer squash, unpeeled, cut lengthwise into thin, spaghetti-like strips

1 1/2 tablespoons Asian peanut satay sauce of choice (page 167)

1 tablespoon tahini

Juice of 1/2 lime (1 tablespoon)

1 teaspoon naturally brewed soy sauce

1 teaspoon freshly grated gingerroot

1/3 cup thinly sliced fresh snow peas

1/3 cup thinly sliced red or orange bell pepper

1 teaspoon white or black sesame seeds, toasted

2 tablespoons fresh cilantro leaves

Zucchini acts like noodles to make this main dish fresh and filling. But it's the flavors, textures, and beauty that'll bring you back to this recipe again and again. Use one zucchini and one yellow summer squash for the best looking results. Make it with steak, and it's a marvelous meal in one.

1. Add the zucchini to a 2-quart microwave-safe dish.

2. Stir together the satay sauce, tahini, lime juice, soy sauce, and ginger in a small bowl until smooth. Pour the sauce over the zucchini and toss to coat.

3. Cover the dish with unbleached parchment paper and microwave on high until the vegetables are done, about 4 minutes (for al dente) to 5 minutes (for softened). Remove from the microwave and let stand, covered, for 5 minutes to complete the cooking process.

4. Add the snow peas and bell pepper, toss to combine, and adjust seasoning. Sprinkle with the sesame seeds and cilantro, and serve immediately.

WITH POULTRY, FISH, OR MEAT

For one serving (full recipe): Before preparing the recipe, grill a 2-ounce piece of grass-fed beef tenderloin or boneless sirloin until medium-rare, about 1 1/2 minutes per side. Let stand for at least 5 minutes. Cut into long, extra-thin slices. Sprinkle with a smidgen of sea salt. Toss with the summer squash noodles, snow peas, and bell pepper in step 4.

Satay Sauce

For Satay Zucchini Noodles, you can use your favorite store-bought satay sauce, your own recipe, or this:

Jackie's Peanut Satay Sauce

Makes 9 servings: 2 tablespoons each

1/2 cup creamy natural peanut butter

1/3 cup plain unsweetened coconut milk beverage or almond milk (not coconut milk)

2 tablespoons unsweetened applesauce or apple-peach sauce

Juice of 1 lime (2 tablespoons)

1 tablespoon naturally brewed soy sauce

1 1/2 teaspoons freshly grated gingerroot

1 teaspoon toasted sesame oil

1/8 teaspoon dried hot pepper flakes, or to taste

Add the peanut butter, coconut milk beverage, applesauce, lime juice, soy sauce, ginger, sesame oil, and hot pepper flakes to a blender and purée. Enjoy as a dipping sauce for satay, a basting sauce for grilled chicken or tofu, or a dressing for noodles and salads. Makes 1 1/8 cups.

Exchanges/Food Choices: 1/2 Carbohydrate, 1 1/2 Fat
90 calories, 70 calories from fat, 8g total fat, 2g saturated fat, 0g trans fat, 0mg cholesterol, 170mg sodium, 100mg potassium, 4g total carbohydrate, 1g dietary fiber, 2g sugars, 4g protein, 50mg phosphorus

without
Exchanges/Food Choices: 1 Carbohydrate, 3 Vegetable, 3 Fat
260 calories, 140 calories from fat, 16g total fat, 2.5g saturated fat, 0g trans fat, 0mg cholesterol, 460mg sodium, 1300mg potassium, 24g total carbohydrate, 8g dietary fiber, 12g sugars, 12g protein, 320mg phosphorus

with
Exchanges/Food Choices: 1 Carbohydrate, 3 Vegetable, 2 Lean Meat, 2 Fat
330 calories, 160 calories from fat, 18g total fat, 3g saturated fat, 0g trans fat, 30mg cholesterol, 570mg sodium, 1490mg potassium, 24g total carbohydrate, 8g dietary fiber, 12g sugars, 25g protein, 440mg phosphorus

Creamy Eggplant Korma

Makes 4 servings: 1 3/4 cups each

2 teaspoons canola or unrefined
  peanut oil

1 medium red onion, finely diced

1 (15-ounce) can no-salt-added tomato
  sauce, divided

1/2 teaspoon sea salt, divided

1 large (1 1/2-pound) eggplant,
  unpeeled, cut into 1/2-inch cubes

3 large garlic cloves, minced

2 teaspoons freshly grated gingerroot

2 tablespoons no-salt-added creamy
  peanut or almond butter

1 tablespoon garam masala curry paste
  or other red curry paste

2 teaspoons ground coriander

1/4 cup finely chopped dried
  unsulphured apricots or black
  seedless raisins

1 1/4 cups plain unsweetened almond
  milk or coconut milk beverage
  (not coconut milk)

1 pint grape tomatoes

3 tablespoons sliced natural almonds,
  toasted

1/4 cup chopped fresh cilantro

If you're in the mood for tasty comfort food, this recipe is made for you. It has distinct Indian flavors, but is balanced enough for nearly every palate. The creamy korma is full of wonderful textures, including crunchiness from the almonds, along with pops of color from the tomato and cilantro. You'll love how the tomatoes burst in your mouth. Enjoy it as is or served over steamed brown basmati rice or whole-wheat couscous.

1. Heat the oil in a large, deep, nonstick skillet or Dutch oven over medium heat. Add the onion, 1/4 cup tomato sauce, and 1/4 teaspoon salt, and sauté until the onion is softened, about 8 minutes. Add the eggplant, garlic, and ginger, and cook while stirring until the eggplant is heated through, about 3 minutes.

2. Add the peanut butter, curry paste, coriander, and the remaining tomato sauce, and cook while stirring until the mixture is well combined and steamy hot, about 5 minutes. Add the dried apricots, almond milk, and the remaining 1/4 teaspoon salt, and bring to a boil over high heat.

3. Reduce heat to medium-low and simmer, covered, until the eggplant is fully cooked, about 10 minutes, stirring a couple times during the simmering process. Stir in the grape tomatoes and simmer, covered, until the tomatoes are heated through, about 5 minutes. Adjust seasoning.

4. Ladle the korma into individual bowls, sprinkle with the almonds and cilantro, and serve.

{ WITH POULTRY, FISH, OR MEAT }

One serving: Transfer 1 3/4 cups korma to a small saucepan immediately after stirring in the grape tomatoes in step 3. Add 1 ounce shredded or cubed rotisserie or roasted chicken white meat to the korma in the small saucepan and simmer, covered, for about 5 minutes. Adjust seasoning.

Full recipe: Stir 4 ounces shredded or cubed rotisserie or roasted chicken white meat into the korma along with the grape tomatoes in step 3. Adjust seasoning.

without
Exchanges/Food Choices: 1 1/2 Carbohydrate, 4 Vegetable, 2 Fat
240 calories, 90 calories from fat, 10g total fat, 1g saturated fat, 0g trans fat, 0mg cholesterol, 490mg sodium, 1090mg potassium, 31g total carbohydrate, 9g dietary fiber, 18g sugars, 8g protein, 150mg phosphorus

with
Exchanges/Food Choices: 1 1/2 Carbohydrate, 4 Vegetable, 1 Lean Meat, 2 Fat
280 calories, 100 calories from fat, 11g total fat, 1.5g saturated fat, 0g trans fat, 25mg cholesterol, 590mg sodium, 1170mg potassium, 31g total carbohydrate, 9g dietary fiber, 18g sugars, 16g protein, 220mg phosphorus

Grilled Eggplant Steak

Makes 2 servings: 2 steaks each

1 large eggplant, cut into 4 thick slices lengthwise (about 6 ounces per slice)

2 1/2 teaspoons extra-virgin olive oil

1/2 teaspoon freshly ground black pepper, or to taste

1/4 teaspoon sea salt, or to taste

Pinch ground cinnamon

2 teaspoons pine nuts, toasted

1 tablespoon small fresh mint leaves

2 lemon wedges

Usually, "steak" refers to a cut of meat. Now the term "steak" can apply to so many foods, including these thick, hearty slices of grilled eggplant. They're succulent and fill up the plate even more than a traditional serving of steak. Savor their Middle Eastern flair along with a protein-rich appetizer or side, like beans, edamame, or hummus.

1. Prepare an outdoor or indoor grill. Lightly brush the eggplant with the oil using a silicone brush. Sprinkle with the pepper, salt, and cinnamon.

2. Grill over direct medium-high heat until fully cooked through and rich grill marks form, about 6–7 minutes per side. Adjust seasoning.

3. Transfer to 2 plates and sprinkle with the pine nuts and mint. Serve with the lemon wedges on the side.

{ WITH POULTRY, FISH, OR MEAT }

One serving: Heat 1 teaspoon extra-virgin olive oil in a small, nonstick skillet over medium heat. Add 1/2 cup finely chopped red onion and 1 1/2 ounces lean, ground, grass-fed beef sirloin, and sauté until the beef is done and onion is softened, about 5 minutes. Add 1/2 cup low-sodium vegetable broth, 1/4 cup marinara sauce of choice (page 191), and 1/8 teaspoon ground cinnamon, and bring to a boil over high heat. Reduce heat to low and simmer, uncovered, until desired consistency, about 8–10 minutes. Ladle over one serving of the eggplant steaks in step 3 before sprinkling with the pine nuts and mint.

Full recipe: Heat 2 teaspoons extra-virgin olive oil in a large, nonstick skillet over medium heat. Add 1 cup finely chopped red onion and 3 ounces lean, ground, grass-fed beef sirloin and sauté until the beef is done and onion is softened, about 5 minutes. Add 1 cup low-sodium vegetable broth, 1/2 cup marinara sauce of choice (page 191), and 1/4 teaspoon ground cinnamon, and bring to a boil over high heat. Reduce heat to low and simmer, uncovered, until desired consistency, about 8–10 minutes. Ladle over the eggplant steaks in step 3 before sprinkling with the pine nuts and mint.

without
Exchanges/Food Choices: 3 1/2 Vegetable, 1 1/2 Fat
160 calories, 70 calories from fat, 8g total fat, 1g saturated fat, 0g trans fat, 0mg cholesterol, 300mg sodium, 820mg potassium, 22g total carbohydrate, 10g dietary fiber, 11g sugars, 4g protein, 100mg phosphorus

with
Exchanges/Food Choices: 1/2 Starch, 5 Vegetable, 1 Lean Meat, 3 Fat
320 calories, 130 calories from fat, 15g total fat, 2.4g saturated fat, 0g trans fat, 20mg cholesterol, 570mg sodium, 1290mg potassium, 36g total carbohydrate, 15g dietary fiber, 15g sugars, 14g protein, 240mg phosphorus

Roasted Cauliflower Steak with Mushroom Sauce

Makes 2 servings: 1 steak with 1/2 cup sauce each

2 (1-inch-thick) whole slices from a medium head cauliflower (about 6 ounces per slice)

2 1/2 teaspoons extra-virgin olive oil, divided

1 teaspoon minced fresh rosemary, divided

1/4 teaspoon freshly ground black pepper, divided

1/8 teaspoon sea salt, or to taste

1 1/2 cups thinly sliced crimini mushrooms (4 ounces)

1/2 cup marinara sauce of choice (page 191)

1/4 cup low-sodium vegetable broth or water

1/8 teaspoon dried hot pepper flakes, or to taste

2 teaspoons pine nuts, toasted

I adore roasted cauliflower, especially when served in a steak-like fashion. The cauliflower makes an enticing and generously sized entrée. Herbaceous rosemary laces both the cauliflower and the sauce, and the spiced mushroom-marinara sauce makes this an extra-hearty bite. It's a perfect dish for couples.

1. Preheat the oven to 425°F. Brush the cauliflower "steaks" with 1 1/2 teaspoons oil and arrange on a baking sheet. Roast until lightly caramelized and the cauliflower florets are cooked through, about 20 minutes. Gently flip over each "steak," sprinkle with 1/2 teaspoon minced rosemary, 1/8 teaspoon black pepper, and the salt, and roast until well caramelized and the cauliflower stems are cooked through, about 12 minutes. Adjust seasoning.

2. Meanwhile, heat the remaining 1 teaspoon oil in a small saucepan over medium heat. Add the mushrooms and the remaining 1/2 teaspoon rosemary and 1/8 teaspoon black pepper, and sauté until the mushrooms are softened, about 5 minutes. Add the marinara sauce, broth, and hot pepper flakes, and bring to a boil over medium-high heat. Reduce heat to low and simmer, covered, until desired consistency, about 8 minutes. Adjust seasoning.

3. Top each cauliflower steak with the sauce and pine nuts, and serve as an entrée.

WITH POULTRY, FISH, OR MEAT

One serving: When the mushroom sauce begins to simmer in step 2, spritz a small, nonstick skillet with cooking spray. Add 2 ounces ground turkey (about 94% lean) and a smidgen of sea salt over medium-high heat, and sauté until fully cooked and crumbled, about 2 minutes. Transfer 1/2 cup mushroom sauce to the turkey in the skillet, reduce heat to low, and simmer, covered, until desired consistency, about 6 minutes.

Full recipe: Add 4 ounces crumbled, uncooked ground turkey (about 94% lean) and a pinch of sea salt along with the mushrooms in step 2.

without
Exchanges/Food Choices: 3 Vegetable, 2 Fat
150 calories, 80 calories from fat, 10g total fat, 1g saturated fat, 0g trans fat, 0mg cholesterol, 470mg sodium, 710mg potassium, 15g total carbohydrate, 5g dietary fiber, 8g sugars, 6g protein, 160mg phosphorus

with
Exchanges/Food Choices: 3 Vegetable, 2 Lean Meat, 2 Fat
240 calories, 130 calories from fat, 14g total fat, 2.5g saturated fat, 0g trans fat, 45mg cholesterol, 580mg sodium, 830mg potassium, 15g total carbohydrate, 5g dietary fiber, 8g sugars, 16g protein, 270mg phosphorus

Creating Cauliflower "Steaks"

With a chef's knife, slice down from the top of the cauliflower head down through the stem end. Use the largest center slices as "steaks." Reserve the remaining cauliflower for other recipes, such as Chimichurri Hummus and Cauliflower Wrap (page 138) and "Fettuccine" Primavera (page 198).

Tzatziki Tofu and Vegetable Kebabs

Makes 4 servings: 1 tofu skewer, 1 zucchini skewer,
and 1 bell pepper skewer each

1 (14-ounce) package extra-firm tofu, drained and squeezed of excess liquid, cut into 16 cubes

2 medium zucchini, cut into 6 (1-inch) cubes each

1 1/2 cups tzatziki sauce of choice (page 175), divided

1 large red bell pepper, cut into about 32 pieces

1/2 teaspoon sea salt, or to taste

1/4 teaspoon freshly ground black pepper, or to taste

2 scallions, green and white parts, thinly sliced on the diagonal

Take veggies, skewer, and grill! Pair with tangy Greek-style yogurt sauce, and it is extra delicious. Enjoy these grilled veggie skewers as is, over steamed brown basmati rice, or served in whole-grain pita.

1. Add the tofu to a medium bowl. Add the zucchini to a large bowl. Add 3/4 cup tzatziki sauce to each bowl and gently toss to coat. Let marinate for about 1 hour.

2. Prepare an outdoor or indoor grill. Thread the tofu onto 4 (8 × 10-inch) reusable or water-soaked bamboo skewers, the zucchini onto 4 other skewers, and the (nonmarinated) bell pepper onto 4 other skewers. Reserve the tzatziki used for marinating the zucchini; it can be reused since it wasn't in contact with raw poultry, fish, or meat.

3. Grill the kebabs over direct medium-high heat until cooked through and rich grill marks form, about 12 minutes, turning only as needed. (Note: Carefully flip the tofu skewers with the help of a spatula only once.) Add the salt and pepper to taste.

4. Arrange the grilled kebabs onto a platter or individual plates. Sprinkle with the scallions, and serve the reserved tzatziki sauce (about 1/2 cup) with the kebabs, or just with the tofu.

One serving: Use 11 1/2 ounces tofu (12 cubes) for the main recipe. Then, in a small bowl, separately marinate 6 (1/2-ounce) cubes of chicken breast in 3 tablespoons tzatziki sauce in step 1. Thread onto 1 skewer and grill next to or after the tofu and vegetables. Do not reuse any of this tzatziki sauce during grilling or at serving.

Full recipe: Instead of the 14 ounces tofu, marinate 24 (1/2-ounce) cubes of chicken breast in tzatziki sauce in step 1. Do not reuse any of this tzatziki sauce during grilling or at serving.

without
Exchanges/Food Choices: 2 Vegetable, 1 Medium-Fat Meat, 1 Fat
160 calories, 80 calories from fat, 9g total fat, 1g saturated fat, 0g trans fat, 0mg cholesterol, 370mg sodium, 570mg potassium, 10g total carbohydrate, 3g dietary fiber, 6g sugars, 14g protein, 220mg phosphorus

with
Exchanges/Food Choices: 2 Vegetable, 2 Lean Meat, 1 Fat
160 calories, 45 calories from fat, 5g total fat, 1g saturated fat, 0g trans fat, 50mg cholesterol, 380mg sodium, 580mg potassium, 8g total carbohydrate, 2g dietary fiber, 5g sugars, 21g protein, 210mg phosphorus

Tzatziki Sauce

For Tzatziki Tofu and Vegetable Kebabs, you can use your favorite store-bought tzatziki sauce, your own recipe, or this:

Jackie's Minty Tzatziki Sauce

Makes 12 servings: 2 tablespoons each

1/3 cup chopped unpeeled English cucumber
2 large garlic cloves, peeled
1 1/4 cups plain fat-free Greek yogurt
2 tablespoons extra-virgin olive oil

Juice of 1/2 small lemon (1 tablespoon)
1/2 teaspoon sea salt, or to taste
1/4 teaspoon freshly ground black pepper, or to taste
1 tablespoon finely chopped fresh mint

Add the cucumber and garlic to a food processor. Cover and pulse until finely chopped. Add the yogurt, oil, lemon juice, salt, and pepper, and blend until well combined. Transfer the yogurt mixture to a medium bowl. Stir in the mint, and serve. Makes 1 1/2 cups.

Exchanges/Food Choices: 1/2 Fat
35 calories, 20 calories from fat, 2.5g total fat, 0g saturated fat, 0g trans fat, 0mg cholesterol, 105mg sodium, 40mg potassium, 1g total carbohydrate, 0g dietary fiber, 1g sugars, 2g protein, 30mg phosphorus

Kung Pao Peppers and Tofu

Makes 4 servings: 1 1/4 cups each

1 tablespoon canola or peanut oil

3 large bell peppers, various colors, diced

1 small Serrano pepper, with some seeds, thinly sliced

1 tablespoon freshly grated gingerroot

3 large garlic cloves, very thinly sliced

3/4 cup Asian Stir-Fry Sauce (page 177)

4 scallions, green and white parts, sliced on the diagonal

3 tablespoons coarsely chopped salted dry-roasted peanuts

6 ounces Asian-flavored ready-to-eat baked tofu, diced

This Kung Pao sure packs a pow. It's rich in color, texture, and flavor. The Asian baked tofu makes it a bona fide entrée. But the best part for some may be that once you prep the ingredients, it takes just 5 minutes from wok to table. Enjoy over buckwheat soba noodles or steamed brown rice. Serve with extra brown rice vinegar or soy sauce on the side for additional pep, if you like.

1. Heat the oil in a wok or large, deep skillet over high heat. Carefully add the bell peppers, Serrano pepper, ginger, and garlic, and stir-fry until the bell peppers are al dente, about 3 minutes. Add the stir-fry sauce and scallions, and stir-fry until the sauce is slightly thickened, about 30 seconds. Add the peanuts and stir-fry until the sauce is thickened, about 30 seconds.

2. Immediately stir in the tofu until heated through, about 30 seconds, and serve.

Poaching Shrimp

Add 1 quart water, a few lemon slices, and, if desired, a pinch of salt to a large saucepan, and bring to a boil over high heat. Add the shrimp, reduce heat to medium-low, cover, and cook until the shrimp is opaque in the center, about 3–4 minutes for medium shrimp. Drain. If not using right away, add to a bowl of icy water to halt the cooking process, then immediately drain again.

{ WITH POULTRY, FISH, OR MEAT }

One serving: Transfer about 1 cup stir-fry to a serving bowl at the end of step 1. Stir 8 warm, poached, cleaned, deveined medium shrimp into the serving instead of tofu. Use 4 1/2 ounces instead of 6 ounces tofu for the main recipe.

Full recipe: Stir 32 poached, cleaned, deveined medium shrimp into the stir-fry along with the peanuts in step 1. Do not add tofu.

without
Exchanges/Food Choices: 2 Vegetable,
1 Medium-Fat Meat, 2 Fat
230 calories, 120 calories from fat, 14g total fat,
2g saturated fat, 0g trans fat, 0mg cholesterol,
460mg sodium, 500mg potassium, 16g total
carbohydrate, 4g dietary fiber, 6g sugars,
14g protein, 200mg phosphorus

with
Exchanges/Food Choices: 1 Carbohydrate,
1 Vegetable, 1 Lean Meat, 2 Fat
180 calories, 90 calories from fat, 10g total fat,
1g saturated fat, 0g trans fat, 60mg cholesterol,
550mg sodium, 430mg potassium, 14g total
carbohydrate, 3g dietary fiber, 6g sugars,
11g protein, 180mg phosphorus

Asian Stir-Fry Sauce

Makes 4 servings: 3 tablespoons each

1/2 cup low-sodium vegetable broth
2 tablespoons no-sugar-added applesauce or apple-peach sauce
1 tablespoon brown rice vinegar
1 tablespoon naturally brewed soy sauce
1 1/2 teaspoons toasted sesame oil
2 teaspoons cornstarch

Whisk together the broth, applesauce, vinegar, soy sauce, oil, and cornstarch in a liquid measuring cup until smooth. Makes 3/4 cup. Use in Kung Pao Peppers and Tofu.

Exchanges/Food Choices: 1/2 Fat
30 calories, 15 calories from fat, 2g total fat, 0g saturated fat, 0g trans fat, 250mg sodium,
10mg potassium, 3g total carbohydrate, 0g dietary fiber, 1g sugars, 1g protein, 0mg phosphorus

Caribbean Black Bean Bowl

Makes 4 servings: 1 1/3 cups each

1 tablespoon canola or peanut oil

1 large sweet potato, scrubbed, unpeeled, finely diced

2 large green bell peppers, diced

2 teaspoons freshly grated gingerroot

2 large garlic cloves, very thinly sliced

3 scallions, thinly sliced, green and white parts separated

1 (15-ounce) can black beans, gently rinsed and drained (1 1/2 cups)

1 cup small grape tomatoes

1/2 cup low-sodium vegetable broth

1/2 cup light coconut milk

1/2 teaspoon sea salt, or to taste

1/8 teaspoon ground cayenne pepper or black pepper, or to taste

Pinch ground cinnamon or allspice, or to taste

2 tablespoons coarsely chopped roasted unsalted peanuts

You'll prepare this recipe like a stir-fry, but it has nothing to do with Chinese takeout! All of the tastes and textures of this vivid recipe work so well together. The coconut milk creates richness and a distinct Caribbean accent. Once you prep the ingredients, this "stir-fry" is so quick to fix. Serve as is or try over steamed brown jasmine rice for a complete meal in a bowl that tastes rather tropical.

1. Heat the oil in a wok or large skillet over high heat. Add the sweet potato and stir-fry for 2 minutes. Add the bell peppers and stir-fry until the sweet potato and bell peppers are caramelized, about 5 minutes. Add the ginger, garlic, and white part of the scallions and stir-fry for 30 seconds. Add the beans, tomatoes, broth, coconut milk, salt, cayenne, and cinnamon, and stir-fry until the excess liquid has evaporated yet mixture is still very moist, about 2 1/2–3 minutes. Stir in the green part of the scallions. Remove from heat and adjust seasoning.

2. Transfer to a large serving bowl or individual bowls, sprinkle with the peanuts, and serve.

{ WITH POULTRY, FISH, OR MEAT }

One serving: Finely dice 1/2 ounce ready-to-eat smoked pork loin. Transfer 1 1/3 cups stir-fry at the beginning of step 2 to a separate dish and stir in the pork.

Full recipe: Finely dice 2 ounces ready-to-eat smoked pork loin. Add to the stir-fry along with the beans in step 1.

without
Exchanges/Food Choices: 2 Starch, 1 Vegetable, 1 Fat
230 calories, 70 calories from fat, 8g total fat, 2g saturated fat, 0g trans fat, 0mg cholesterol, 460mg sodium, 850mg potassium, 34g total carbohydrate, 9g dietary fiber, 11g sugars, 8g protein, 190mg phosphorus

with
Exchanges/Food Choices: 2 Starch, 1 Vegetable, 1/2 Lean Meat, 1 Fat
250 calories, 80 calories from fat, 8g total fat, 2g saturated fat, 0g trans fat, 10mg cholesterol, 590mg sodium, 890mg potassium, 34g total carbohydrate, 9g dietary fiber, 11g sugars, 11g protein, 220mg phosphorus

Garnet Yam Stack

Makes 4 servings: 1 stack each

2 large (10-ounce) garnet sweet
   potatoes ("red yams"), cut into
   1/2-inch thick slices crosswise

1 (14-ounce) package extra-firm tofu,
   drained and squeezed of excess
   liquid, cut in half lengthwise,
   then each half cut into 8 slices
   crosswise

2/3 cup low-sodium vegetable broth,
   divided

3 tablespoons aged balsamic vinegar

1 tablespoon extra-virgin olive oil

3 large garlic cloves, minced

1/4 teaspoon + 1/8 teaspoon sea salt,
   or to taste

1 cup marinara sauce of choice
   (page 191)

1/3 cup crumbled goat cheese
   (1 1/3 ounces)

1/4 teaspoon dried hot pepper flakes,
   or to taste

28 large fresh basil leaves

Here's one of the most show-stopping entrées you'll ever make. On a bed of creamy goat-cheese marinara sauce with a sunset-orange hue, you'll form a towering stack with alternating layers of roasted garnet red sweet potato, caramelized tofu, and fresh basil leaves. It's especially eye-appealing with grill markings on the tofu. It's a taste-bud temptress, too.

1. Add the sweet potato slices (use only the largest 16 slices) and the 16 tofu slices into a 9 × 13-inch dish. Whisk together 1/3 cup broth, the vinegar, oil, garlic, and 1/4 teaspoon salt in a liquid measuring cup. Pour over the sweet potato and tofu slices, and let marinate for about 1 hour, turning with tongs a couple times so the slices get evenly marinated.

2. Preheat the oven to 450°F. Arrange the sweet potato and tofu slices in an even layer on a large baking sheet lined with unbleached parchment paper. Roast until the sweet potato and tofu slices are lightly caramelized and the sweet potato is fully cooked, about 30 minutes. Sprinkle with the remaining 1/8 teaspoon salt. (Alternatively, while roasting the sweet potatoes, grill the tofu over medium-high heat until rich grill marks form, about 2 1/2–3 minutes per side.)

3. Meanwhile, add the marinara sauce, goat cheese, hot pepper flakes, and the remaining 1/3 cup broth to a small saucepan over medium-high heat. Bring to a boil while stirring. Remove from heat. (Note: If you used a chunky rather than smooth marinara, quickly purée the sauce in a blender or with an immersion blender for a velvety consistency.)

4. Ladle about 1/3 cup goat-cheese marinara onto each of 4 individual plates. On top of the sauce, carefully arrange in alternating stacked layers the sweet potato, tofu, and fresh basil leaves. If desired, use a bamboo skewer to help each stack stand upright, and serve with additional balsamic vinegar on the side.

{ WITH POULTRY, FISH, OR MEAT }

One serving: Prepare 1 ounce of a fully cooked sweet Italian poultry sausage link according to package directions. Slice into "coins." Serve around one of the stacks, on the goat-cheese marinara sauce.

Full recipe: Prepare 4 ounces fully cooked sweet Italian poultry sausage links according to package directions. Slice into "coins." Serve around each of the stacks, on the goat-cheese marinara sauce.

without
Exchanges/Food Choices: 2 Starch, 1 Lean Meat, 1 Fat
260 calories, 90 calories from fat, 10g total fat, 2g saturated fat, 0g trans fat, 5mg cholesterol, 420mg sodium, 780mg potassium, 27g total carbohydrate, 4g dietary fiber, 9g sugars, 15g protein, 230mg phosphorus

with
Exchanges/Food Choices: 2 Starch, 2 Lean Meat, 1 Fat
290 calories, 110 calories from fat, 13g total fat, 3g saturated fat, 0g trans fat, 30mg cholesterol, 580mg sodium, 830mg potassium, 28g total carbohydrate, 5g dietary fiber, 9g sugars, 20g protein, 290mg phosphorus

Mint Pesto Couscous and Peas

Makes 4 servings: 1 cup each

1/3 cup roasted unsalted shelled pistachios

2 large garlic cloves, peeled

1 cup packed fresh mint leaves + 4 fresh mint sprigs

3 ounces drained soft tofu (1/2 scant cup crumbled)

1 1/2 cups low-sodium vegetable broth, divided

2 teaspoons fresh lemon juice

1/8 teaspoon + 1/2 teaspoon sea salt, or to taste

2 tablespoons extra-virgin olive oil

3/4 cup whole-wheat couscous

1 1/2 cups frozen thawed peas

Couscous is served here as a super-moist, fragrant, and comforting entrée. Fresh mint-pistachio pesto gives it unique taste, and the peas provide a lovely contrasting texture along with a burst of veggie nutrition. Form it using a measuring cup or ring mold to make it an attention-grabbing focal point on the plate.

1. Add the pistachios and garlic to a food processor. Cover and pulse until the garlic is finely chopped. Add the mint leaves, tofu, 1/4 cup broth, the lemon juice, and 1/8 teaspoon salt. Cover, and pulse until just combined. Add the oil and purée to desired consistency. Set aside.

2. Bring the remaining 1 1/4 cups broth and the remaining 1/2 teaspoon salt to a boil in a small saucepan over high heat. Stir in the couscous and peas. Immediately cover and remove from heat. Let stand for 7 minutes, covered, to finish the cooking process. Stir in the mint-pistachio pesto until well combined, and adjust seasoning.

3. Transfer to individual bowls, or form on individual plates using a measuring cup or ring mold. Garnish with the mint sprigs, and serve.

{ WITH POULTRY, FISH, OR MEAT }

One serving: Arrange 5 small, ready-to-eat, cooked shrimp on top of one of the servings of couscous in step 3, before garnishing with the mint sprigs.

Full recipe: Add 20 small, chilled, ready-to-eat, cooked shrimp (thawed, if frozen) along with couscous and peas in step 2. Alternatively, arrange the prepared shrimp on top of each serving before garnishing with the mint sprigs in step 3.

without
Exchanges/Food Choices: 2 1/2 Starch,
1 Vegetable, 2 1/2 Fat
310 calories, 110 calories from fat, 13g total fat,
1.5g saturated fat, 0g trans fat, 0mg cholesterol,
450mg sodium, 250mg potassium, 40g total
carbohydrate, 9g dietary fiber, 5g sugars,
12g protein, 150mg phosphorus

with
Exchanges/Food Choices: 2 1/2 Starch,
1 Vegetable, 2 Lean Meat, 1 Fat
330 calories, 120 calories from fat, 13g total fat,
1.5g saturated fat, 0g trans fat, 30mg cholesterol,
590mg sodium, 280mg potassium, 41g total
carbohydrate, 9g dietary fiber, 5g sugars,
15g protein, 210mg phosphorus

Cajun Veggies, Smoked Tofu, and Couscous

Makes 4 servings: 1 cup vegetable mixture
and 3/4 cup couscous each

1 tablespoon extra-virgin olive oil

1 medium red onion, diced

1 large green bell pepper, diced

1 cup finely chopped cauliflower

1 tablespoon red wine vinegar

1/4 teaspoon sea salt, or to taste

3 large garlic cloves, finely chopped

3/4 cup low-sodium vegetable broth

2 large vine-ripened or beefsteak tomatoes, seeds removed and diced

1 teaspoon fresh thyme or oregano leaves + 4 fresh thyme or oregano sprigs

1/2 teaspoon chili powder

1/4 teaspoon freshly ground black pepper, or to taste

1/8 teaspoon ground cayenne pepper, or to taste

6 ounces smoked or savory baked tofu, cut into 1/3-inch cubes

3 cups Scallion-Herb Couscous (page 185) or prepared whole-wheat couscous of choice, warm

Get ready for a bowlful of flavor fulfillment. The veggies are stew-like with kicked-up excitement from Cajun culinary influences. The tofu adds a surprise smokiness to lend another tasty layer. It's transformed into a comforting meal by serving it over couscous.

1. Heat the oil in a large, deep, nonstick skillet or Dutch oven over medium-high heat. Add the onion, bell pepper, cauliflower, vinegar, and salt, and sauté until the onion begins to caramelize, about 8 minutes. Add the garlic and sauté for 30 seconds. Stir in the broth, tomatoes, thyme leaves, chili powder, black pepper, and cayenne. Cook until the cauliflower is fully cooked, gently stirring occasionally, until no excess liquid remains and mixture is very moist, about 8 minutes. Stir in the tofu, reduce heat to low, and cook, covered, to allow the tofu to absorb flavors, about 8 minutes. Adjust seasoning.

2. Add the couscous to individual bowls or a platter. Top with the tofu-vegetable mixture, garnish with the thyme sprigs, and serve.

{ WITH POULTRY, FISH, OR MEAT }

One serving: Prepare an outdoor or indoor grill. Insert 4 (1/2-ounce) cubes of chicken or turkey breast onto a reusable or water-soaked bamboo skewer and sprinkle with 1/8 teaspoon Cajun seasoning. Alternatively, sprinkle the seasoning on a 2-ounce portion of farm-raised catfish fillet. Grill over direct medium-high heat for 4–5 minutes per side. Place atop one of the servings before garnishing.

Full recipe: Prepare an outdoor or indoor grill. Insert 16 (1/2-ounce) cubes of chicken or turkey breast onto 4 reusable or water-soaked bamboo skewers and sprinkle with 1/2 teaspoon Cajun seasoning. Alternatively, sprinkle the seasoning on one 8-ounce farm-raised catfish fillet. Grill over direct medium-high heat for 4–5 minutes per side. Place atop each serving before garnishing.

without
Exchanges/Food Choices: 2 1/2 Starch, 1 Vegetable, 1 Medium-Fat Meat
270 calories, 60 calories from fat, 7g total fat, 1g saturated fat, 0g trans fat, 0mg cholesterol, 440mg sodium, 560mg potassium, 42g total carbohydrate, 9g dietary fiber, 9g sugars, 14g protein, 210mg phosphorus

with
Exchanges/Food Choices: 2 Starch, 1 Vegetable, 3 Lean Meat
330 calories, 70 calories from fat, 8g total fat, 1.5g saturated fat, 0g trans fat, 30mg cholesterol, 570mg sodium, 660mg potassium, 42g total carbohydrate, 9g dietary fiber, 9g sugars, 25g protein, 290mg phosphorus

Scallion-Herb Couscous

Makes 4 servings: 3/4 cup each

3/4 cup (uncooked) whole-wheat couscous
1 scallion, green and white parts, minced

1/4 teaspoon sea salt, or to taste
2 tablespoons chopped fresh flat-leaf parsley

Bring 1 1/4 cups cold water to a boil over high heat in a small saucepan. Stir in the couscous, scallion, and salt. Cover and turn off the heat. Let stand for 7 minutes. Stir in the parsley while fluffing with a fork. Makes 3 cups. Enjoy in Cajun Veggies, Smoked Tofu, and Couscous or as a simple side dish.

Exchanges/Food Choices: 2 Starch
130 calories, 5 calories from fat, 0g total fat, 0g saturated fat, 0mg cholesterol, 150mg sodium, 70mg potassium, 28g total carbohydrate, 5g dietary fiber, 1g sugars, 5g protein, 60mg phosphorus

BB&B Fajitas

Makes 6 servings: 1 fajita each

1/2 cup plain fat-free Greek yogurt

2 tablespoons chopped fresh cilantro

Juice of 1/2 lime (1 tablespoon), divided

1 (15-ounce) can pinto beans, gently rinsed and drained (1 1/2 cups)

2/3 cup mild pico de gallo (fresh chunky salsa)

1 tablespoon peanut or canola oil

1 medium white onion, halved and sliced

1 small jalapeño pepper, with some seeds, halved lengthwise and thinly sliced crosswise

2 large red or green bell peppers, or one of each, thinly sliced

2 cups broccoli slaw (shredded mixture of broccoli, carrots, and red cabbage)

1/2 teaspoon ground cumin

1/4 teaspoon sea salt, or to taste

1/2 cup guacamole of choice (page 159)

6 soft taco-size whole-wheat or other whole-grain tortillas, warm

The three B's in the title are for the savory stars of the recipe—beans, bell peppers, and broccoli. But the title isn't the only thing fun about these fajitas! Everyone gets to fill up their own tortilla DIY (do-it-yourself)-style. Your tortilla will be quite full, so, if you prefer, wrap it up and enjoy burrito-style.

1. Stir together the yogurt, cilantro, and 1 teaspoon lime juice in a small bowl, and set aside.

2. Stir together the beans and pico de gallo in a small saucepan. Cover and place over low heat to warm.

3. Meanwhile, heat the oil in a wok or large, deep skillet over medium-high heat. Add the onion and jalapeño, and sauté until the onion is slightly softened, about 2 minutes. Increase heat to high, add the bell peppers, broccoli slaw, cumin, salt, and the remaining 2 teaspoons lime juice, and stir-fry until all vegetables are cooked through and the onion is lightly caramelized, about 4 minutes. Transfer to a serving dish and adjust seasoning.

4. Serve the vegetable mixture (4 cups), bean mixture (2 cups), yogurt mixture (2/3 cup), and guacamole (1/2 cup) family-style with the tortillas.

{ WITH POULTRY, FISH, OR MEAT }

One serving: Grill a 1 1/2-ounce portion of lean, grass-fed flank steak or U.S. Atlantic or Pacific yellowfin tuna steak over direct medium-high heat until medium-rare, about 2 minutes per side for beef or 3 minutes per side for tuna. Let stand at least 5 minutes. Very thinly slice against the grain. Sprinkle with a pinch of freshly ground black pepper and dash of sea salt. Provide in a separate dish along with the other ingredients in step 4.

Full recipe: Grill a 9-ounce portion of lean, grass-fed flank steak or U.S. Atlantic or Pacific yellowfin tuna steak over direct medium-high heat until medium-rare, about 2–2 1/2 minutes per side for beef or 3–3 1/2 minutes per side for tuna. Let stand at least 5 minutes. Very thinly slice against the grain. Sprinkle with 1/4 teaspoon freshly ground black pepper and a pinch of sea salt. Provide in a separate dish along with the other ingredients in step 4.

without
Exchanges/Food Choices: 2 Starch, 3 Vegetable, 2 Fat
290 calories, 70 calories from fat, 8g total fat, 0.5g saturated fat, 0g trans fat, 0mg cholesterol, 550mg sodium, 610mg potassium, 45g total carbohydrate, 9g dietary fiber, 8g sugars, 11g protein, 230mg phosphorus

with
Exchanges/Food Choices: 2 Starch, 3 Vegetable, 1 Lean Meat, 1 1/2 Fat
360 calories, 100 calories from fat, 11g total fat, 2g saturated fat, 0g trans fat, 25mg cholesterol, 600mg sodium, 710mg potassium, 45g total carbohydrate, 9g dietary fiber, 8g sugars, 20g protein, 300mg phosphorus

Roasted Vegetable Enchilada Bake

Makes 6 servings: 1/6 casserole each

2 teaspoons canola or unrefined peanut oil

1 large sweet onion, diced

1 1/4 cups mild or medium tomatillo salsa (salsa verde) of choice, divided

12 ounces crimini or white button mushrooms, sliced

1 fresh Poblano pepper, chopped

5 cups packed fresh baby spinach (5 ounces)

1 (15-ounce) can pinto beans, gently rinsed and drained (1 1/2 cups)

3 tablespoons chopped fresh cilantro

1 teaspoon finely chopped fresh oregano leaves

1/2 teaspoon ground cumin

1/4 teaspoon sea salt, or to taste

12 (6-inch) corn tortillas

1/2 cup shredded Monterey Jack or pepper jack cheese (2 ounces)

If you're a fan of Mexican cuisine, you'll definitely give a thumbs-up to this rather luscious casserole-style dish. The tomatillo salsa gives it delightful tang, and the Poblano pepper and pinto beans provide rich body. The mushrooms impart meatiness, and the Monterey Jack offers cheesiness, of course. The distinctive tastes of cilantro, oregano, and cumin make this recipe unforgettable. If you have calories to spare, take your portion over the top by topping with a dollop of guacamole (page 159).

1. Preheat the oven to 400°F.

2. Heat the oil in a large, deep, nonstick skillet over medium-high heat. Add the onion and 1/4 cup salsa, and sauté until the onion is softened, about 8 minutes. Add the mushrooms and Poblano pepper, and sauté until the mushrooms are softened, about 8 minutes. Stir in the spinach, and toss until just wilted, about 1 minute. Add the beans, cilantro, oregano, cumin, and salt, and sauté until fully combined and heated through, about 1 minute. Adjust seasoning.

3. Spread 1/2 cup salsa into a 9 × 13-inch baking dish. Arrange 6 tortillas to cover the bottom of the dish. Evenly top with half of the vegetable mixture. Arrange the remaining 6 tortillas on top. Sprinkle with 1/4 cup salsa. Evenly top with the remaining vegetable mixture. Sprinkle with the cheese. Bake until fully cooked through and the cheese is melted, about 20 minutes. Sprinkle with the remaining 1/4 cup salsa.

4. Cut the casserole into 6 portions, and serve.

WITH POULTRY, FISH, OR MEAT

One serving: Sprinkle 1 ounce finely cubed roasted pork tenderloin or shredded roasted pork loin onto a one-sixth section of the casserole before sprinkling with the cheese in step 3.

Full recipe: Sprinkle 6 ounces finely cubed roasted pork tenderloin or shredded roasted pork loin onto the casserole after arranging the remaining 6 tortillas in step 3.

without
Exchanges/Food Choices: 2 Starch, 2 Vegetable, 1 Fat
270 calories, 60 calories from fat, 7g total fat, 2.5g saturated fat, 0g trans fat, 10mg cholesterol, 430mg sodium, 860mg potassium, 43g total carbohydrate, 9g dietary fiber, 7g sugars, 13g protein, 350mg phosphorus

with
Exchanges/Food Choices: 2 Starch, 2 Vegetable, 1 Lean Meat, 1 Fat
310 calories, 70 calories from fat, 7g total fat, 2.5g saturated fat, 0g trans fat, 30mg cholesterol, 450mg sodium, 980mg potassium, 43g total carbohydrate, 9g dietary fiber, 7g sugars, 20g protein, 420mg phosphorus

Roasted Asparagus Parmigiana with Pasta

Makes 4 servings: 8 asparagus spears
and about 3/4 cup pasta each

32 green or white asparagus spears,
ends trimmed

1 tablespoon canola or extra-virgin
olive oil

1 cup marinara sauce of choice
(page 191)

2 tablespoons low-sodium vegetable
broth or water

1 teaspoon finely chopped fresh
rosemary (optional)

2 tablespoons minced fresh chives

1/4 teaspoon freshly ground black
pepper, or to taste

1/8 teaspoon sea salt, or to taste

1/3 cup part-skim mozzarella cheese
(1 1/2 ounces)

2 teaspoons grated Parmigiano-
Reggiano or other Parmesan
cheese

2 garlic cloves, thinly sliced

5 ounces whole-wheat spinach or
other whole-grain linguine or
spaghetti

2 tablespoons finely chopped fresh
basil

"Parmigiana" refers to a dish that's prepared or served with Parmesan cheese. Besides that, today's Parmigiana doesn't have to contain fried veal, chicken, or even eggplant. Here, I've chosen asparagus for a deliciously different twist. Roasted, and served over spinach pasta while incorporating plenty of herbs, this Italian-style dish will be a savory treat.

1. Preheat the oven to 425°F. Place the asparagus onto 2 large baking pans. Drizzle with the oil and toss to coat. Arrange the asparagus spears in alternating fashion. Roast until the asparagus is lightly caramelized on the bottom, yet still firm, about 8 minutes. Meanwhile, stir together the marinara sauce, vegetable broth, and rosemary (if using) in a liquid measuring cup or small bowl; set aside.

2. Flip each piece of asparagus over. Separate the asparagus into 4 compact sets of 8 asparagus each. Sprinkle each set with the chives, pepper, salt, marinara sauce mixture, mozzarella, Parmigiano-Reggiano, and garlic. Roast until the cheese is bubbly and golden brown and the asparagus is fully cooked, about 15–18 minutes. Adjust seasoning.

3. Meanwhile, prepare the pasta according to package directions. Drain, reserving 1/4 cup cooking liquid. Toss the pasta with the basil and reserved cooking liquid.

4. Transfer the pasta to four separate plates or pasta bowls; arrange each set of asparagus on top of the pasta, and serve.

{ WITH POULTRY, FISH, OR MEAT }

One serving: Top one set of the asparagus with 1/2 thawed, frozen ready-to-heat breaded chicken patty before topping with the marinara sauce mixture in step 2. If desired, transfer to a separate baking pan.

Full recipe: Top each set of the asparagus with 1/2 thawed, frozen ready-to-heat breaded chicken patty before topping with the marinara sauce mixture in step 2. (You'll need 2 chicken patties total.)

without
Exchanges/Food Choices: 2 Starch, 1 Vegetable, 1 1/2 fat
250 calories, 70 calories from fat, 7g total fat, 1.5g saturated fat, 0g trans fat, 5mg cholesterol, 450mg sodium, 550mg potassium, 37g total carbohydrate, 8g dietary fiber, 6g sugars, 12g protein, 230mg phosphorus

with
Exchanges/Food Choices: 3 Starch, 1 Vegetable, 1 Lean Meat, 2 Fat
370 calories, 120 calories from fat, 13g total fat, 3.5g saturated fat, 0g trans fat, 30mg cholesterol, 550mg sodium, 690mg potassium, 45g total carbohydrate, 8g dietary fiber, 6g sugars, 20g protein, 350mg phosphorus

Marinara Sauce

Some recipes suggest using "marinara sauce of choice." You can use your favorite store-bought variety, your own recipe, or mine:

Jackie's Marinara Sauce

Makes 8 servings: 1/2 cup each

2 teaspoons extra-virgin olive oil
1 medium yellow onion, diced
1 tablespoon red wine vinegar
1/4 teaspoon sea salt, or to taste
2 large garlic cloves, minced

1 (28-ounce) can crushed roasted tomatoes
1/3 cup low-sodium vegetable broth or water
1/4 cup chopped fresh flat-leaf parsley
1/8 teaspoon dried hot pepper flakes
2 tablespoons thinly sliced fresh basil

Heat the oil in a large saucepan over medium heat. Add the onion, vinegar, and salt, and sauté until the onion is softened, about 8 minutes. Add the garlic and sauté until fragrant, about 1 minute. Stir in the tomatoes, broth, parsley, and hot pepper flakes, increase heat to high, and bring to a boil. Cover, reduce heat to low, and simmer to allow flavors to develop, about 18 minutes. Stir in the basil, adjust seasoning, and serve. Makes 4 cups.

Exchanges/Food Choices: 2 Vegetable
50 calories, 15 calories from fat, 1.5g total fat, 0g saturated fat, 0g trans fat, 0mg cholesterol, 210mg sodium, 330mg potassium, 9g total carbohydrate, 2g dietary fiber, 5g sugars, 2g protein, 40mg phosphorus

Eggplant and Spaghetti Marinara

1 1/2 cups marinara sauce of choice (page 191)

1 tablespoon extra-virgin olive oil

1 medium (1-pound) eggplant, cut into 1/2-inch cubes

2 garlic cloves, minced

1 teaspoon aged balsamic vinegar

1/8 teaspoon sea salt, or to taste

5 ounces whole-wheat or other whole-grain spaghetti

2 tablespoons thinly sliced fresh basil leaves or 2 fresh basil sprigs

You can turn spaghetti with jarred sauce into something rather special. Garlicky sautéed eggplant is all it takes to glam up this stand-by and make it more satisfying. The finish of fresh basil creates cuisine delight.

1. Bring the marinara sauce to a boil over high heat in a small saucepan. Reduce heat to low, cover, and keep warm.

2. Heat the oil in a large, nonstick skillet over medium heat. Add the eggplant, garlic, vinegar, and salt, and sauté until the eggplant is fully softened, about 18 minutes. Adjust seasoning.

3. Meanwhile, cook the pasta according to package directions in a large saucepan. Drain the pasta, reserving 1/2 cup cooking liquid. Return the pasta to the large saucepan and toss with the eggplant mixture, marinara sauce, and desired amount of the reserved cooking liquid. Adjust seasoning.

4. Divide the pasta among 4 plates or pasta bowls. Top with the basil, and serve.

{ WITH POULTRY, FISH, OR MEAT }

One serving: Heat 1/2 teaspoon extra-virgin olive oil in a small, nonstick skillet over medium heat. Add 1 1/2 ounces ground turkey (about 94% lean) and sauté until well done, about 2 1/2 minutes. Add a smidgen of sea salt and dried hot pepper flakes to taste. Toss with 1 1/4 cups pasta at the end of step 3. Alternatively, stir a minced anchovy into one serving of the pasta.

Full recipe: Heat 2 teaspoons extra-virgin olive oil in a small, nonstick skillet over medium heat. Add 6 ounces ground turkey (about 94% lean) and sauté until well done, about 3 minutes. Add 1/8 teaspoon each sea salt and dried hot pepper flakes to taste. Stir into the marinara sauce while keeping warm in step 1. Alternatively, stir 4 minced anchovies into the sauce.

without
Exchanges/Food Choices: 2 1/2 Starch, 1 Vegetable, 1 Fat
230 calories, 50 calories from fat, 6g total fat, 1g saturated fat, 0g trans fat, 0mg cholesterol, 470mg sodium, 450mg potassium, 40g total carbohydrate, 8g dietary fiber, 9g sugars, 7g protein, 130mg phosphorus

with
Exchanges/Food Choices: 2 1/2 Starch, 1 Vegetable, 1 Lean Meat, 1 1/2 fat
310 calories, 100 calories from fat, 11g total fat, 2g saturated fat, 0g trans fat, 35mg cholesterol, 570mg sodium, 540mg potassium, 41g total carbohydrate, 8g dietary fiber, 9g sugars, 15g protein, 220mg phosphorus

Noodles, Shapes, and Orzo

♦ I based the nutrition analysis on the use of no added salt to the pasta water while cooking. It'll help you keep your sodium intake in better check by leaving it out, even if the cooking directions on the pasta package suggest adding salt. However, if you prefer to keep the salt, just bear it in mind when you plan your meals for the day, so you stay within a healthful total daily sodium allowance.

♦ For preparation time, always stick to the low end of any range given. For example, cook for 9 minutes if the package says to cook for 9–11 minutes. This will mean your pasta will be al dente (just cooked through). That suggests it will have a more enjoyable texture and a lower glycemic index than if you cooked pasta till fully softened. That's helpful for anyone trying to manage a healthy blood glucose level.

♦ A unique way to prepare pasta is by using my eco-friendly technique, "lid cooking." If you're the energy-saving type, try it. Basically, bring water to a boil and stir in the pasta. Bring back to a boil, cover, and turn off the heat. If using an electric stove, remove from the burner. Then let it "lid cook" (cook without heat with the lid on) for the same amount of time suggested on the package, again using the low end of any time range given. That's it!

Orecchiette and Kale with Pecorino Romano

Makes 4 servings: 1 3/4 cups each

7 ounces dry whole-wheat or other whole-grain orecchiette or farfalle

1 tablespoon extra-virgin olive oil

2 large garlic cloves, thinly sliced

1/8 teaspoon dried hot pepper flakes, or to taste

1 pound green kale or lacinato ("dinosaur") kale, roughly chopped, stems trimmed

1 tablespoon dried currants or minced black seedless raisins

Juice and zest of 1/2 small lemon (1 tablespoon juice)

1/4 teaspoon + 1/8 teaspoon sea salt, or to taste

1/3 cup freshly grated Pecorino Romano or Parmigiano-Reggiano cheese (1 1/4 ounces)

1/2 teaspoon freshly ground black pepper, or to taste

You'll be using either cute little ear-shaped pasta or bow-tie shaped pasta for this recipe. The veggies are the center of attention, though, rather than just a garnish for this pasta. Here, the aim was to use about twice the amount of veggies as pasta. Putting the spotlight on kale makes each serving so much bigger and more satisfying. Best of all, it's delicious.

1. Cook the orecchiette according to package directions.

2. Meanwhile, heat the oil in a Dutch oven over medium-high heat. Add the garlic and hot pepper flakes, and sauté until fragrant, about 30 seconds. Add the kale and currants, and sauté until the kale is wilted, about 5 minutes. Add the lemon juice and salt, toss to combine, cover, and set aside.

3. Drain the pasta, reserving 1/2 cup cooking liquid. Add the pasta, cheese, black pepper, and desired amount of the reserved pasta cooking liquid to the Dutch oven with the kale, and toss using tongs. Adjust seasoning.

4. Divide the pasta among individual plates or pasta bowls, sprinkle with the lemon zest, and serve immediately.

{ WITH POULTRY, FISH, OR MEAT }

One serving: Prepare 3/4 ounce of a fully cooked andouille or spicy poultry sausage link. Slice into very thin "coins" and toss into one of the servings of pasta in step 4.

Full recipe: Prepare a 3-ounce link of fully cooked andouille or spicy poultry sausage. Slice into very thin "coins" and toss into the kale in the Dutch oven in step 3.

without
Exchanges/Food Choices: 2 1/2 Starch,
1 Vegetable, 1 1/2 Fat
270 calories, 60 calories from fat, 7g total fat,
2.5g saturated fat, 0g trans fat, 5mg cholesterol,
400mg sodium, 350mg potassium, 45g total
carbohydrate, 6g dietary fiber, 4g sugars,
12g protein, 160mg phosphorus

with
Exchanges/Food Choices: 2 Starch, 2 Vegetable,
1 Medium-Fat Meat, 1 fat
310 calories, 80 calories from fat, 9g total fat,
3g saturated fat, 0g trans fat, 25mg cholesterol,
510mg sodium, 390mg potassium, 45g total
carbohydrate, 7g dietary fiber, 4g sugars,
15g protein, 200mg phosphorus

Creamy Mediterranean Radiatore

Makes 6 servings: 1 rounded cup each

1 (15-ounce) can chickpeas (garbanzo beans), gently rinsed and drained, divided (1 1/2 cups)

1 1/4 cups marinara sauce of choice (page 191)

1/2 cup low-sodium vegetable broth

1 tablespoon lemon juice + zest of 1 lemon

1 teaspoon minced fresh rosemary

8 ounces dry whole-wheat or other whole-grain radiatore, cavatelli, or rotini

5 cups packed fresh baby spinach or finely chopped Swiss chard leaves (5 ounces)

1/4 teaspoon + 1/8 teaspoon sea salt, or to taste

1/4 teaspoon freshly ground black pepper, or to taste

2 1/2 tablespoons pine nuts, toasted

You'll be amazed at the creaminess of this pasta dish. It's truly decadent without needing a drop of cream. Chickpeas provide the velvetiness of the sauce. Baby spinach creates extra interest—and extra veggies, of course. And the Mediterranean accents of fragrant rosemary, zesty lemon, and toasty pine nuts take the taste of this comforting pasta over the top.

1. Add 1 cup chickpeas, the marinara sauce, broth, lemon juice, and rosemary to a blender. Cover and purée until velvety smooth, at least 2 minutes. Pour the creamy marinara sauce into a medium saucepan. Bring to a boil over high heat. Cover, reduce heat to low, and simmer for about 12 minutes.

2. Meanwhile, cook the radiatore in a large saucepan according to package directions until al dente. Drain the pasta.

3. Return the pasta to the large, dry saucepan over medium heat. Add the creamy marinara sauce and the remaining chickpeas, and toss to coat. Add the spinach and salt, and toss to coat while cooking until the spinach just wilts, about 1 1/2 minutes. Adjust seasoning.

4. Transfer the pasta to a large serving bowl or individual bowls, sprinkle with the pepper, lemon zest, and pine nuts, and serve.

{ WITH POULTRY, FISH, OR MEAT }

One serving: Rub or brush 1 1/2 ounces boneless, skinless chicken breast with 1/2 teaspoon extra-virgin olive oil. Grill or pan-grill until well done. Sprinkle with a pinch of freshly ground black pepper and smidgen of sea salt. Dice the chicken, then sprinkle onto 1 rounded cup pasta in step 4, before sprinkling the pasta with the pepper, lemon zest, and pine nuts.

Full recipe: Rub or brush 9 ounces boneless, skinless chicken breast with 1 tablespoon extra-virgin olive oil. Grill or pan-grill until well done. Sprinkle with 1/2 teaspoon freshly ground black pepper and 1/4 teaspoon sea salt. Dice the chicken and stir into the pasta along with the spinach in step 3.

without
Exchanges/Food Choices: 3 Starch, 1 Fat
250 calories, 45 calories from fat, 5g total fat,
0g saturated fat, 0g trans fat, 0mg cholesterol,
490mg sodium, 380mg potassium, 43g total
carbohydrate, 7g dietary fiber, 6g sugars,
11g protein, 140mg phosphorus

with
Exchanges/Food Choices: 3 Starch, 1 Lean Meat,
1 Fat
310 calories, 70 calories from fat, 8g total fat,
1g saturated fat, 0g trans fat, 25mg cholesterol,
600mg sodium, 450mg potassium, 43g total
carbohydrate, 7g dietary fiber, 6g sugars,
19g protein, 210mg phosphorus

"Fettuccine" Primavera

1/4 cup low-sodium vegetable broth

1 teaspoon extra-virgin olive oil

1/4 teaspoon sea salt, divided

14 asparagus spears, cut into 1/2-inch thick pieces on the diagonal, ends trimmed

1 1/4 cups small bite-size cauliflower floret pieces

1 small white or yellow onion, quartered, thinly sliced

1 (8-ounce) package tofu Shirataki fettuccine-shaped noodles

1 1/2 tablespoons basil pesto

1/2 teaspoon lemon zest, or to taste

It's hard to believe that you can have a bowl of pasta with pesto for just 150 calories! But using tofu noodles makes this dreamy dish a reality. The fettuccine-like noodles are kind of funky, in a good way, especially because they're just 20 calories a serving. The roasted veggies make this "pasta" dish hearty, the pesto makes it divine, and the lemon zest atop the primavera creates fragrant zip.

1. Preheat the oven to 450°F. Whisk together the broth, oil, and 1/8 teaspoon salt in a medium bowl. Add the asparagus, cauliflower, and onion, and toss until well coated. Arrange in a single layer onto an unbleached parchment paper–lined large baking sheet and roast until the vegetables are caramelized, about 35 minutes.

2. Meanwhile, drain, rinse, and prepare the noodles according to package directions. Then drain but do not dry the noodles.

3. Toss together the roasted veggies, hot drained noodles, and the remaining 1/8 teaspoon salt in a medium serving bowl. Add the pesto and toss well to coat. Adjust seasoning. Sprinkle with the lemon zest, and serve while warm.

{ WITH POULTRY, FISH, OR MEAT }

One serving: Add 3 large, fresh, wild, dry sea scallops (side muscles removed, rinsed and patted dry) and 1/2 teaspoon extra-virgin olive oil to a small bowl, and toss to coat. Cook on a preheated grill pan over medium-high heat until done, about 2 1/2 minutes per side. Divide the primavera in step 3 into 2 bowls. (Note: Skip the 1/8 teaspoon salt in step 3 or add just a pinch to the serving without the scallops.) Add the scallops onto one of the servings; sprinkle with the lemon zest.

Full recipe: Add 6 large, fresh, wild, dry sea scallops (side muscles removed, rinsed and patted dry) and 1 teaspoon extra-virgin olive oil to a small bowl, and toss to coat. Cook on a preheated grill pan over medium-high heat until done, about 2 1/2 minutes per side. (Note: Do not add the 1/8 teaspoon salt in step 3.) Arrange the scallops atop the primavera in step 3; sprinkle with the lemon zest.

without
Exchanges/Food Choices: 2 Vegetable, 2 Fat
150 calories, 80 calories from fat, 9g total fat,
2g saturated fat, 0g trans fat, 5mg cholesterol,
430mg sodium, 490mg potassium, 14g total
carbohydrate, 6g dietary fiber, 4g sugars,
7g protein, 160mg phosphorus

with
Exchanges/Food Choices: 2 Vegetable,
1 Lean Meat, 2 Fat
200 calories, 100 calories from fat, 11g total fat,
2.5g saturated fat, 0g trans fat, 15mg cholesterol,
470mg sodium, 580mg potassium, 16g total
carbohydrate, 6g dietary fiber, 4g sugars,
12g protein, 310mg phosphorus

Grilled Vegetable Shirataki

Makes 2 servings: 2 cups each

2 large (3-ounce) portabella
mushroom caps

1 large (11-ounce) zucchini, unpeeled,
cut lengthwise into 5 strips

1 pint grape tomatoes

2 teaspoons extra-virgin olive oil

1 garlic clove, creamed or grated

1 (8-ounce) package tofu Shirataki
noodles

1 1/2 teaspoons white balsamic or
aged balsamic vinegar

1/4 cup thinly sliced fresh basil

1/4 teaspoon sea salt, or to taste

1/4 cup shredded part-skim
mozzarella cheese (1 ounce)

In my opinion, the all-time tastiest way to enjoy veggies is straight from the grill. Rather than just giving you a plate of grilled veggies, here you'll get a big bowl mixed with noodles. That means you'll get to savor grilled vegetables as a fully satisfying entrée in addition to keeping calories friendly, thanks especially to the super low-cal tofu Shirataki.

1. Prepare an outdoor or indoor grill. Place the mushroom caps, zucchini, and tomatoes into a large bowl or dish. Drizzle with the oil and toss to coat. Insert the tomatoes onto reusable or water-soaked bamboo skewers.

2. Grill the mushroom caps, zucchini, and tomato skewers over direct medium-high heat until cooked through and grill marks form, about 8 total minutes, flipping only once during cooking. Remove the grape tomatoes from the skewers and gently toss with the garlic in the large bowl. Dice the mushroom caps and zucchini, and add to the tomato mixture. Cover to keep warm.

3. Meanwhile, drain, rinse, and prepare the noodles according to package directions. Then drain but do not dry the noodles.

4. Add the hot drained noodles, vinegar, basil, and salt to the bowl with the vegetables, and gently toss to combine. Adjust seasoning.

5. Transfer to individual bowls, sprinkle with the cheese, and serve.

{ WITH POULTRY, FISH, OR MEAT }

One serving: Skip the 1/4 teaspoon sea salt in step 4. Rather, transfer the Shirataki recipe to individual bowls in step 5 and then sprinkle one serving with 1/8 teaspoon sea salt and add just a pinch of sea salt to this "With Poultry, Fish, or Meat" serving. Finely chop 1/2 ounce thinly sliced prosciutto or American country ham. Sprinkle onto this serving in place of the cheese.

Full recipe: Add 1/8 teaspoon instead of 1/4 teaspoon sea salt to the recipe in step 4. Finely chop 1 ounce thinly sliced prosciutto or American country ham. Sprinkle onto each bowl in place of the cheese in step 5.

without
Exchanges/Food Choices: 3 Vegetable, 2 Fat
170 calories, 80 calories from fat, 9g total fat, 2.5g saturated fat, 0g trans fat, 10mg cholesterol, 420mg sodium, 1090mg potassium, 17g total carbohydrate, 6g dietary fiber, 9g sugars, 10g protein, 220mg phosphorus

with
Exchanges/Food Choices: 3 Vegetable, 1 Lean Meat, 1 Fat
160 calories, 60 calories from fat, 7g total fat, 1.5g saturated fat, 0g trans fat, 10mg cholesterol, 570mg sodium, 1160mg potassium, 17g total carbohydrate, 6g dietary fiber, 9g sugars, 10g protein, 260mg phosphorus

Veggie Chow Fun

Makes 4 servings: 1 1/4 cups each

1/2 cup low-sodium vegetable broth

2 tablespoons naturally brewed soy sauce, or to taste

2 tablespoons no-sugar-added apple or apple-peach sauce

6 ounces dry flat, short, and wide brown rice noodles or broken pad Thai brown rice noodles

2 tablespoons canola or grapeseed oil, divided

3 cups diced eggplant, unpeeled (8 ounces)

1/8 teaspoon sea salt, or to taste

2 large garlic cloves, minced

2 teaspoons freshly grated gingerroot

2 small bunches fresh baby bok choy, thinly sliced (2 3/4 cups sliced)

1 cup oyster mushrooms, separated, or sliced shiitake mushroom caps

4 scallions, green and white parts, thinly sliced on the diagonal

3 tablespoons thinly sliced fresh basil

1 1/2 teaspoons white or black sesame seeds, toasted

Can't beat a bowl of noodles in the wintertime—or anytime, for that matter. This Asian-style bowl is loaded with veggies, including eggplant, baby bok choy, and oyster mushrooms. Full of textures and rich flavor, this chow fun really is fun!

1. Whisk together the broth, soy sauce, and applesauce in a liquid measuring cup. Set aside. Prepare the noodles according to package directions. Rinse under cold water, drain, and transfer to a medium serving bowl. Set aside. (Note: If noodles sit too long and become sticky, rinse and drain again.)

2. Heat 2 teaspoons oil in a wok or large skillet over medium-high heat. Add the eggplant and sauté until just cooked through, about 5 minutes. Transfer to a plate. Set aside.

3. Place the wok over high heat and add 2 teaspoons oil. Add the noodles and stir-fry for 15 seconds. Add half the reserved sauce and the salt, and stir to evenly coat noodles, about 45 seconds. Transfer the noodles back into the serving bowl.

4. Replace the wok over high heat and add the remaining 2 teaspoons oil. Add the garlic and ginger, and stir-fry for 30 seconds. Add the bok choy, mushrooms, scallions, and the reserved eggplant, and stir-fry until all vegetables are fully cooked, about 2 minutes. Return the noodles to the pan along with the remaining reserved sauce, and toss to coat while cooking until fully heated and combined, about 1 minute. Stir in the basil. Adjust seasoning.

5. Transfer to the serving bowl or individual bowls and sprinkle with the sesame seeds. Serve while hot with additional soy sauce on the side, if desired.

WITH POULTRY, FISH, OR MEAT

One serving: Grill or pan-grill a 1 1/2-ounce piece of lean, grass-fed beef tenderloin over direct medium-high heat until medium-rare. Let stand for at least 5 minutes. Very thinly slice against the grain. Immediately stir the beef strips into one serving of the chow fun in step 5 before sprinkling with the sesame seeds.

Full recipe: Add 6 ounces thin, bite-size strips of uncooked, lean, grass-fed beef tenderloin to the wok along with the garlic and ginger in step 4.

without
Exchanges/Food Choices: 2 1/2 Starch, 1 Vegetable, 1 1/2 Fat
270 calories, 80 calories from fat, 9g total fat, 1g saturated fat, 0g trans fat, 0mg cholesterol, 580mg sodium, 390mg potassium, 43g total carbohydrate, 6g dietary fiber, 4g sugars, 7g protein, 70mg phosphorus

with
Exchanges/Food Choices: 2 1/2 Starch, 1 Vegetable, 1 Lean Meat, 2 Fat
330 calories, 100 calories from fat, 11g total fat, 2g saturated fat, 0g trans fat, 25mg cholesterol, 600mg sodium, 500mg potassium, 43g total carbohydrate, 6g dietary fiber, 4g sugars, 15g protein, 140mg phosphorus

Cappellini with Spinach, Canellinis, and Quark

Makes 4 servings: 1 1/4 cups each

4 ounces dry whole-wheat or other whole-grain cappellini pasta

1 tablespoon extra-virgin olive oil, divided

1 (15-ounce) can cannellini or other white beans, gently rinsed and drained (1 1/2 cups)

3 large garlic cloves, thinly sliced

1 tablespoon finely chopped dried fig or other dried fruit bits

8 packed cups fresh baby spinach (8 ounces)

Juice and zest of 1 small lemon (2 tablespoons juice)

1 teaspoon fresh thyme leaves

1/2 teaspoon sea salt, or to taste

1/4 teaspoon dried hot pepper flakes, or to taste

2 ounces quark, at room temperature (1/4 scant cup)

I love pasta for so many reasons, but especially because it's a delicious vehicle in which to enjoy veggies. Not only will you be savoring plenty of spinach in this cappellini (angel hair) recipe, you'll also be boosting your beans to punch up your protein intake. The lemon balances the dish with a fresh brightness. The dollop of quark—European-style fresh cheese curd—completes the pasta with a creamy decadence. But if you can't find quark, sprinkle your serving with feta or goat cheese for a tangy finish instead.

1. Cook the pasta according to package directions. Drain the pasta, transfer to a large bowl, and toss with 1 teaspoon oil. Set aside.

2. Heat the remaining 2 teaspoons oil in a large, deep skillet or wok over medium-high heat. Add the beans and garlic, and sauté until fragrant, about 1 minute. Add the fig, spinach, lemon juice, thyme, salt, hot pepper flakes, and the pasta and cook while tossing with tongs until the spinach is fully wilted, about 2 1/2 minutes. Adjust seasoning.

3. Transfer to individual serving bowls, top each with a dollop of the quark, sprinkle with desired amount of the lemon zest, and serve while warm.

{ WITH POULTRY, FISH, OR MEAT }

One serving: Top one serving of the pasta with a warm mixture of 2 ounces cubed roasted chicken breast, 1/2 teaspoon extra-virgin olive oil, 1 small minced garlic clove (optional), and a smidgen of sea salt.

Full recipe: In a medium bowl, toss together 8 ounces chilled, cubed, roasted chicken breast, 2 teaspoons extra-virgin olive oil, 1 large minced garlic clove (optional), and a pinch of sea salt. Add to the skillet in step 2 after sautéing the beans and garlic slices and before adding the fig.

without

Exchanges/Food Choices: 3 Starch, 1 Fat
270 calories, 50 calories from fat, 6g total fat, 1.5g saturated fat, 0g trans fat, 5mg cholesterol, 520mg sodium, 780mg potassium, 45g total carbohydrate, 11g dietary fiber, 4g sugars, 12g protein, 270mg phosphorus

with

Exchanges/Food Choices: 3 Starch, 3 Lean Meat, 1 Fat
380 calories, 90 calories from fat, 11g total fat, 2g saturated fat, 0g trans fat, 55mg cholesterol, 600mg sodium, 920mg potassium, 45g total carbohydrate, 11g dietary fiber, 4g sugars, 30g protein, 400mg phosphorus

Herbed "Risotto" with Asparagus

Makes 6 servings: 1 cup each

Here's a creamy risotto-style recipe that lets the flavor of nature's best play the lead role, especially the asparagus. Plus, you don't need to stand at the stove and stir continuously as classic arborio risotto requires. Rather, a simplified rice cooking technique is used. The result: a pleasurable dish full of spring garden deliciousness.

1 tablespoon extra-virgin olive oil

1 medium yellow onion, finely chopped

2 teaspoons fresh lemon juice

1 teaspoon sea salt, divided

1 1/2 cups short-grain brown rice

3 1/2 cups low-sodium vegetable broth, divided

1 cup steamed cauliflower floret pieces, warm or at room temperature

1/4 cup fresh mint leaves + 6 fresh mint sprigs

1/4 cup fresh basil leaves

12 asparagus spears, cut into 1/2-inch pieces on the diagonal, ends trimmed

6 sun-dried tomato halves, extra-thinly sliced (do not rehydrate)

1 tablespoon unsalted butter

1 1/2 tablespoons freshly grated Pecorino Romano or Parmigiano-Reggiano cheese

1. Heat the oil in a large saucepan over medium heat. Add the onion, lemon juice, and 1/4 teaspoon salt, and sauté until the onion is softened, about 8 minutes. Stir in the rice, 3 cups broth, and the remaining 3/4 teaspoon salt, increase heat to high, and bring to a boil. Cover, reduce heat to low, and simmer for 30 minutes. The rice will not be fully cooked.

2. Meanwhile, add the steamed cauliflower, mint leaves, basil, and the remaining 1/2 cup broth to a blender. Cover and purée until smooth.

3. Stir the cauliflower-herb purée, asparagus, and sun-dried tomatoes into the rice mixture, cover, and simmer over low heat until the rice is cooked through yet still slightly chewy, about 20 minutes more. Stir in the butter and cheese. Adjust seasoning.

4. Spoon onto individual plates or bowls, top with the mint sprigs, and serve.

{ WITH POULTRY, FISH, OR MEAT }

One serving: Sprinkle 1 ounce warm, diced, rotisserie chicken breast meat on one of the servings before topping with the mint sprigs in step 4.

Full recipe: Stir 6 ounces warm, diced, rotisserie chicken breast meat into the risotto along with the butter and cheese in step 3.

without
Exchanges/Food Choices: 2 1/2 Starch, 1 Vegetable, 1 Fat
250 calories, 50 calories from fat, 6g total fat, 2g saturated fat, 0g trans fat, 5mg cholesterol, 500mg sodium, 320mg potassium, 43g total carbohydrate, 4g dietary fiber, 4g sugars, 6g protein, 170mg phosphorus

with
Exchanges/Food Choices: 2 1/2 Starch, 1 Vegetable, 1 Lean Meat, 1 Fat
290 calories, 60 calories from fat, 7g total fat, 2.5g saturated fat, 0g trans fat, 30mg cholesterol, 600mg sodium, 410mg potassium, 43g total carbohydrate, 4g dietary fiber, 4g sugars, 14g protein, 240mg phosphorus

Edamame and White Veggie "Risotto"

Makes 6 servings: 1 cup each

2 teaspoons extra-virgin olive oil

1 medium white onion, finely chopped

2 teaspoons fresh lemon juice

3/4 teaspoon sea salt, divided

1 1/2 cups short grain brown rice

3 1/2 cups low-sodium vegetable broth, divided

1 cup steamed cauliflower floret pieces, warm or at room temperature

1 cup beech mushrooms or sliced white button mushrooms

1/2 cup frozen shelled edamame

1 tablespoon unsalted butter

2 tablespoons freshly grated Parmigiano-Reggiano or other Parmesan cheese

2 tablespoons thinly sliced fresh basil + 6 fresh basil sprigs

White veggies offer rich nutrition despite their color. So white onion, cauliflower, and white mushrooms are all celebrated here in this non-traditional, rich-tasting risotto dish. Its creaminess actually comes from a purée of cauliflower rather than relying on butter and cheese. This recipe is worthy of a celebration table, too.

1. Heat the oil in a large saucepan over medium heat. Add the onion, lemon juice, and 1/4 teaspoon salt, and sauté until the onion is softened, about 8 minutes. Stir in the rice, 3 cups broth, and the remaining 1/2 teaspoon salt, increase heat to high, and bring to a boil. Cover, reduce heat to low, and simmer for 30 minutes. The rice will not be fully cooked.

2. Meanwhile, add the steamed cauliflower and the remaining 1/2 cup broth to a blender. Cover and purée until smooth.

3. Stir the cauliflower purée and the mushrooms into the rice mixture, cover, and simmer over low heat until the rice is cooked through yet still slightly chewy, about 20 minutes more.

4. Meanwhile, prepare the edamame according to package directions; drain. Stir the edamame, butter, cheese, and sliced basil into the risotto. Adjust seasoning.

5. Spoon onto individual plates or bowls, top with the basil sprigs, and serve.

{ WITH POULTRY, FISH, OR MEAT }

One serving: Add 2 large, fresh, wild, dry sea scallops (side muscles removed, rinsed and patted dry) and 3/4 teaspoon extra-virgin olive oil to a small bowl and toss to coat. Cook on a preheated grill pan over medium-high heat until done, about 2 1/2 minutes per side. Nestle the scallops on top of one of the servings before garnishing with the basil sprig in step 5.

Full recipe: Add 12 large, fresh, wild, dry sea scallops (side muscles removed, rinsed and patted dry) and 1 1/2 tablespoons extra-virgin olive oil to a medium bowl and toss to coat. Cook on a preheated grill pan over medium-high heat until done, about 2 1/2 minutes per side. Nestle 3 scallops on top of each serving before garnishing with the basil sprigs in step 5.

without
Exchanges/Food Choices: 2 1/2 Starch, 1 Vegetable, 1 Fat
250 calories, 50 calories from fat, 6g total fat, 2g saturated fat, 0g trans fat, 5mg cholesterol, 410mg sodium, 290mg potassium, 43g total carbohydrate, 4g dietary fiber, 3g sugars, 7g protein, 180mg phosphorus

with
Exchanges/Food Choices: 2 1/2 Starch, 1 Vegetable, 1/2 Lean Meat, 1 1/2 Fat
310 calories, 90 calories from fat, 10g total fat, 2.5g saturated fat, 0g trans fat, 15mg cholesterol, 520mg sodium, 350mg potassium, 43g total carbohydrate, 4g dietary fiber, 3g sugars, 10g protein, 280mg phosphorus

Lebanese Basmati with Caramelized Onion

Makes 4 servings: 1 1/2 cups each

2 1/2 teaspoons extra-virgin olive oil, divided

1 3/4 cups brown basmati rice, uncooked

4 1/4 cups low-sodium vegetable broth, divided

1 bay leaf

1 teaspoon + 1/8 teaspoon sea salt, or to taste

1 1/4 teaspoons ground cinnamon, or to taste

3/4 cup frozen cut green beans or lima beans, thawed

1 jumbo yellow onion, thinly sliced

1 tablespoon white balsamic vinegar

1/4 cup chopped fresh flat-leaf parsley

1/3 cup pine nuts or slivered almonds, toasted

My mother used to make a Lebanese dish very similar to this rice recipe. It's comforting; the smell of cinnamon permeates the kitchen. The sweet spice is a highlight, so make sure you're using a ground cinnamon that hasn't been sitting in your pantry for years. I hope this nourishing dish becomes comfort food for you, too.

1. Heat 1 1/2 teaspoons oil in a large saucepan over medium heat. Add the rice and stir to coat. Increase heat to high, add 3 3/4 cups broth, the bay leaf, 1 teaspoon salt, and the ground cinnamon, and bring to a boil. Cover, reduce heat to low, and simmer until the rice is nearly cooked, about 35 minutes. Stir in the beans, cover, and continue to cook until the rice and beans are fully cooked, about 10 minutes more.

2. Meanwhile, heat the remaining 1 teaspoon oil in a large, nonstick skillet over medium-high heat. Add the onion, vinegar, and the remaining 1/2 cup broth and 1/8 teaspoon salt, and sauté until the onion is caramelized, about 12 to 15 minutes.

3. Remove the bay leaf from the rice mixture, stir in the caramelized onion, and adjust seasoning.

4. Transfer to individual bowls or a platter and sprinkle with the parsley and pine nuts. Sprinkle with additional cinnamon, if desired, and serve.

WITH POULTRY, FISH, OR MEAT

One serving: Cook 2 ounces lean, ground, grass-fed beef sirloin in a small, nonstick skillet over medium-high heat until done, about 2 minutes. Sprinkle with 1/8 teaspoon freshly ground black pepper, a smidgen of ground cinnamon, and, if desired, sea salt to taste. Before adding the parsley in step 4, sprinkle the beef onto 1 1/2 cups rice mixture

Full recipe: Cook 8 ounces lean, ground, grass-fed beef sirloin in a small, nonstick skillet over medium-high heat until done, about 2 minutes. Sprinkle with 1/2 teaspoon freshly ground black pepper, 1/4 teaspoon ground cinnamon, and, if desired, sea salt to taste. Stir into the rice mixture in step 1 along with the beans.

without
Exchanges/Food Choices: 2 Starch, 1 Vegetable, 1 1/2 Fat
270 calories, 80 calories from fat, 9g total fat, 1g saturated fat, 0g trans fat, 0mg cholesterol, 540mg sodium, 240mg potassium, 45g total carbohydrate, 5g dietary fiber, 4g sugars, 6g protein, 220mg phosphorus

with
Exchanges/Food Choices: 2 Starch, 1 Vegetable, 2 Lean Meat, 1 Fat
340 calories, 100 calories from fat, 11g total fat, 2g saturated fat, 0g trans fat, 30mg cholesterol, 570mg sodium, 390mg potassium, 45g total carbohydrate, 5g dietary fiber, 4g sugars, 17g protein, 310mg phosphorus

Cinnamon

You'll find many recipes contain cinnamon as a spice in *The With or Without Meat Cookbook*. It's considered a "sweet spice," but don't worry, there's no sugar in it. It adds distinctive flavor and often Middle Eastern flair to savory foods.

Bibb and Bean Burrito Bowl

Makes 4 servings: 1 3/4 cups each

- 12 Bibb or Boston lettuce leaves
- 2 1/2 cups drained canned beans, such as a black, pinto, and/or kidney beans
- 2 cups grape tomatoes, quartered lengthwise
- 1 1/4 cups frozen corn, thawed
- 3 scallions, green and white parts, very thinly sliced on the diagonal
- 1/3 cup finely diced Monterey Jack cheese or vegan cheese alternative (1 1/2 ounces)
- 1/4 cup chopped fresh cilantro
- 1/4 teaspoon ground cumin, or to taste
- 1/4 teaspoon chili powder, or to taste
- 1 Hass avocado, peeled, pitted, and diced
- 2/3 cup medium or "hot" tomatillo salsa (salsa verde)
- 1/4 teaspoon sea salt (optional)
- 4 lime wedges

Eating beans every day may help people with type 2 diabetes better manage their blood glucose. So enjoy the health benefits of this inviting meal-in-a-bowl. And enjoy all of its vivid colors, Mexican-inspired flavors, and lovely textures with a fork. The bowl is made from Bibb lettuce, so it's literally an edible bowl! But if you like, use the Bibb leaves to eat some of the bean mixture burrito-style. Any way you choose to eat it, it's muy delicioso.

1. Divide the lettuce leaves among 4 dinner plates or pasta bowls, loosely forming a "bowl" with the leaves.

2. Stir together the beans, tomatoes, corn, scallions, cheese, cilantro, cumin, and chili powder in a medium bowl. Add the avocado, salsa, and salt (if using), and gently stir just to combine. Adjust seasoning.

3. Evenly divide the bean mixture among the 4 lettuce "bowls," and serve with the lime wedges on the side.

WITH POULTRY, FISH, OR MEAT

One serving: Prepare an outdoor or indoor grill. Grill a 2-ounce portion of pork tenderloin or barramundi fillet over direct medium-high heat until medium-well done, about 2–3 minutes per side. Let stand at least 5 minutes. Dice, toss with 1 teaspoon tomatillo salsa, and toss onto one of the "bowls" just before serving in step 3.

Full recipe: Prepare an outdoor or indoor grill. Grill an 8-ounce portion of pork tenderloin or barramundi fillet over direct medium-high heat until medium-well done, about 3–4 minutes per side. Let stand at least 5 minutes. Dice, toss with 1 tablespoon + 1 teaspoon tomatillo salsa, and divide among the "bowls" just before serving in step 3.

without
Exchanges/Food Choices: 2 Starch, 2 Vegetable, 1 1/2 Fat
300 calories, 90 calories from fat, 10g total fat, 3g saturated fat, 0g trans fat, 10mg cholesterol, 550mg sodium, 1070mg potassium, 44g total carbohydrate, 11g dietary fiber, 11g sugars, 13g protein, 300mg phosphorus

with
Exchanges/Food Choices: 2 Starch, 2 Vegetable, 2 Lean Meat, 1 Fat
360 calories, 100 calories from fat, 11g total fat, 3.5g saturated fat, 0g trans fat, 40mg cholesterol, 580mg sodium, 1240mg potassium, 44g total carbohydrate, 11g dietary fiber, 11g sugars, 24g protein, 400mg phosphorus

CHAPTER 7

sides

Saucy Mushrooms

Makes 4 servings: 3/4 cup each

1 tablespoon extra-virgin olive oil

1/2 cup finely chopped sweet onion

1 1/2 pounds sliced mushroom mixture (8 cups)

1 teaspoon minced fresh rosemary or thyme leaves

1/3 cup low-sodium vegetable broth

1 teaspoon naturally brewed soy sauce

1/4 teaspoon sea salt, or to taste

1/2 teaspoon freshly ground black pepper, or to taste

If you want to try a new mushroom variety, this recipe would be my pick for preparing one. Mix up a selection, such as maitake, oyster, and beech, for best results. Then serve this stew-like recipe with its warm waft of fresh rosemary as a succulent side dish. Try it ladled over grains, grits, or Purée of Cauliflower (page 226) if you wish.

1. Heat the oil in a wok or large, deep skillet over medium-high heat. Add the onion, mushrooms, rosemary, broth, and soy sauce, and sauté until the onion and mushrooms are fully softened, about 10 minutes.

2. Add the salt and pepper. Adjust seasoning, and serve.

WITH POULTRY, FISH, OR MEAT

One serving: Dice 1/2 ounce lean, uncured Canadian bacon. Heat in a separate nonstick skillet over medium-high heat until lightly browned, about 1 1/2 minutes. Transfer 3 servings (2 1/4 cups) of the mushroom mixture to a serving bowl at the end of step 2. Stir the Canadian bacon into the remaining 3/4 cup mushroom mixture.

Full recipe: Dice 2 ounces lean, uncured Canadian bacon. Heat in a separate nonstick skillet over medium-high heat until lightly browned, about 1 1/2 minutes. Stir into the mushroom mixture before adding the salt and pepper in step 2.

without
Exchanges/Food Choices: 1 1/2 Vegetable, 1 Fat
70 calories, 30 calories from fat, 3.5g total fat, 0.5g saturated fat, 0g trans fat, 0mg cholesterol, 240mg sodium, 670mg potassium, 8g total carbohydrate, 1g dietary fiber, 4g sugars, 4g protein, 180mg phosphorus

with
Exchanges/Food Choices: 1 1/2 Vegetable, 1 Lean Meat, 1/2 Fat
100 calories, 40 calories from fat, 5g total fat, 1g saturated fat, 0g trans fat, 10mg cholesterol, 460mg sodium, 730mg potassium, 8g total carbohydrate, 1g dietary fiber, 4g sugars, 7g protein, 220mg phosphorus

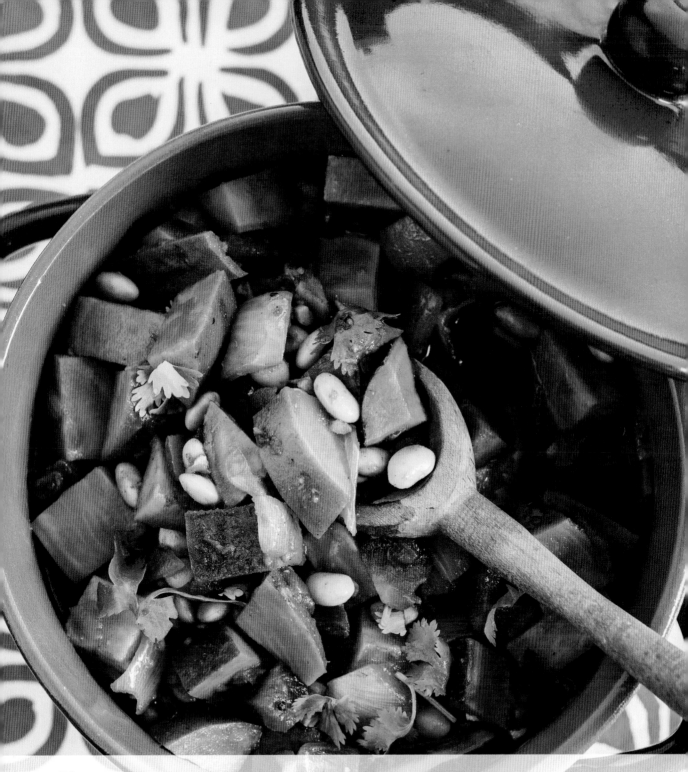

Indian Sweet Potato–Edamame Stew, p. 124

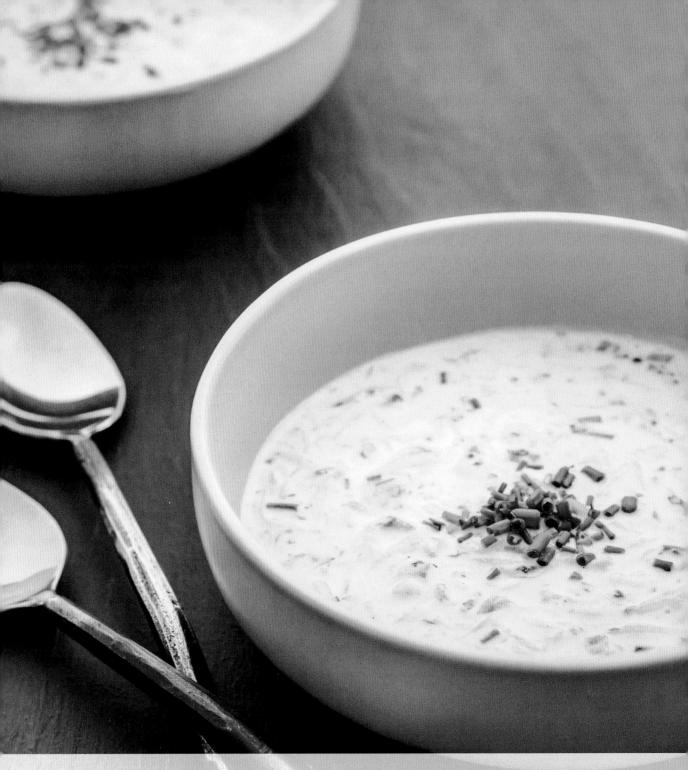

Chilled Persian Cucumber Soup with Chives, p. 134

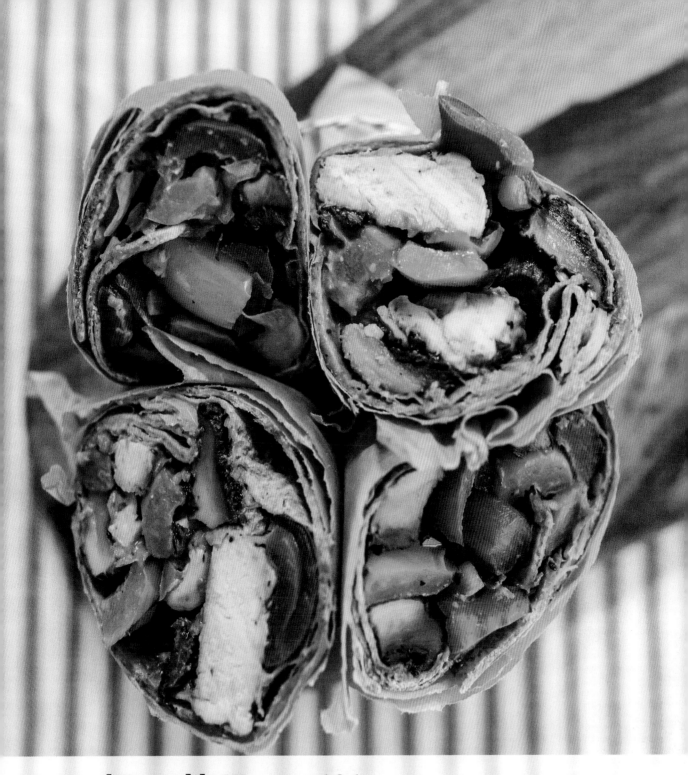

Roasted Vegetable Wrap, p. 136

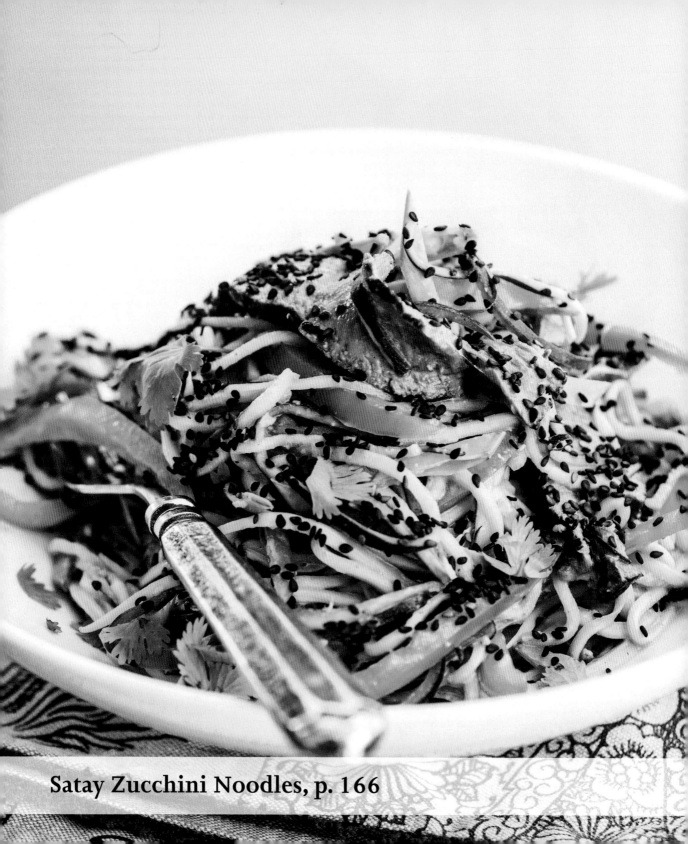

Satay Zucchini Noodles, p. 166

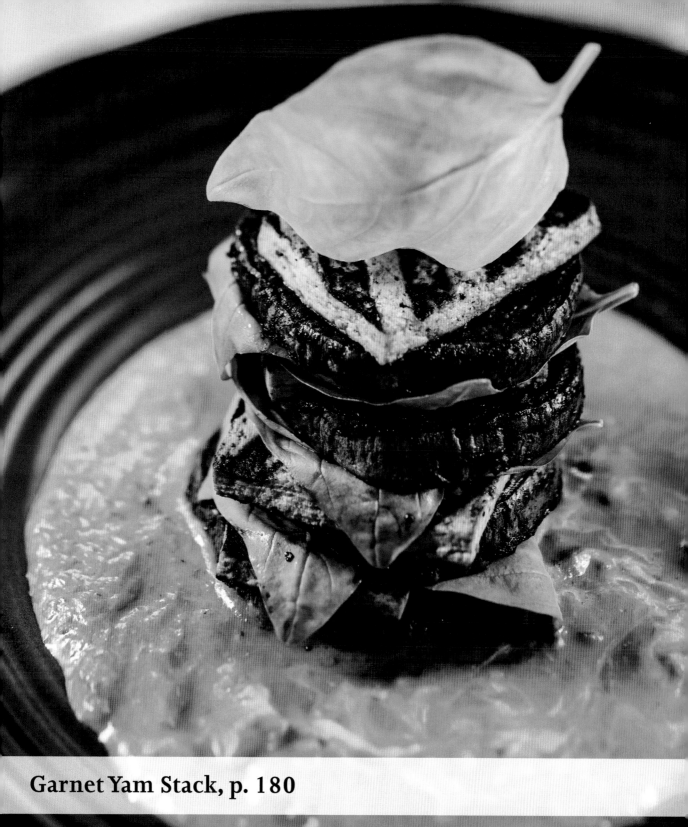

Garnet Yam Stack, p. 180

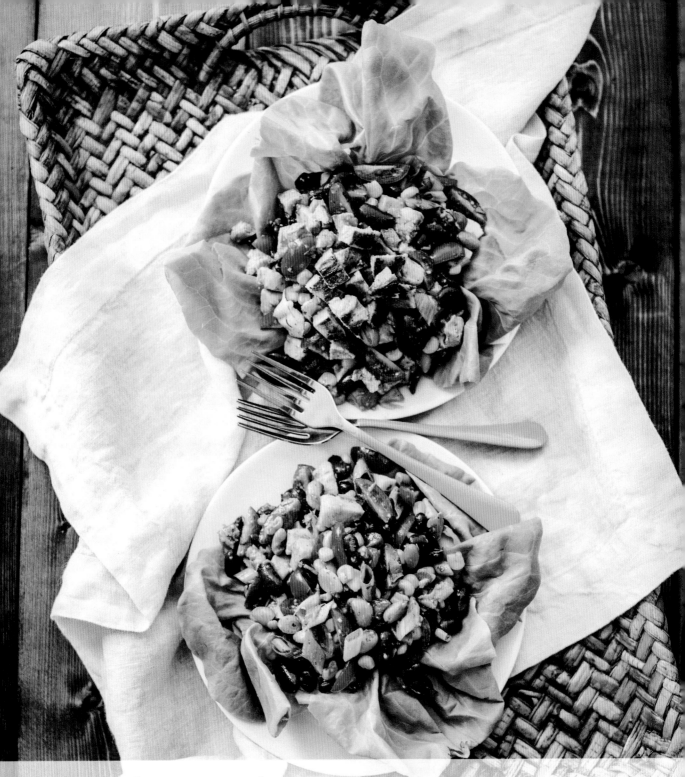

Bibb and Bean Burrito Bowl, p. 212

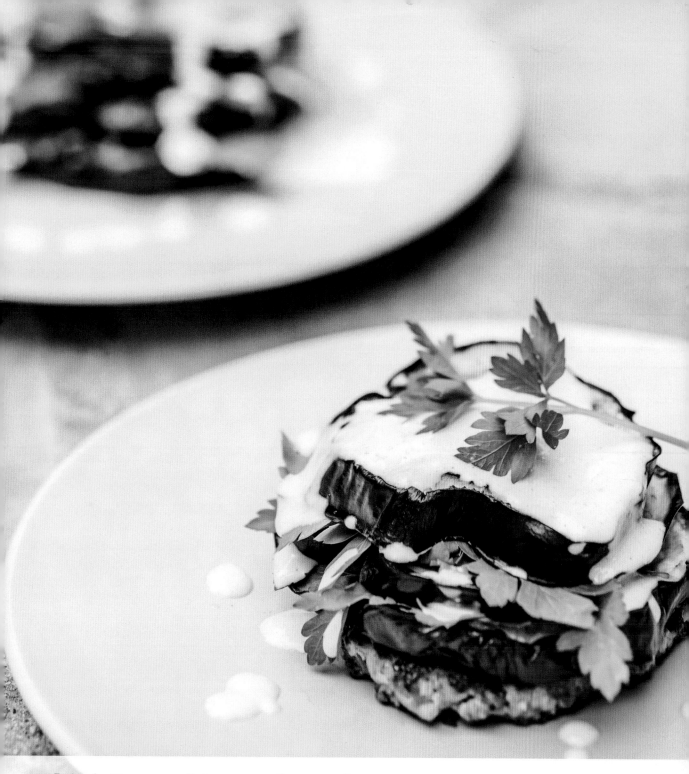

Tahini-Dressed Roasted Eggplant, p. 228

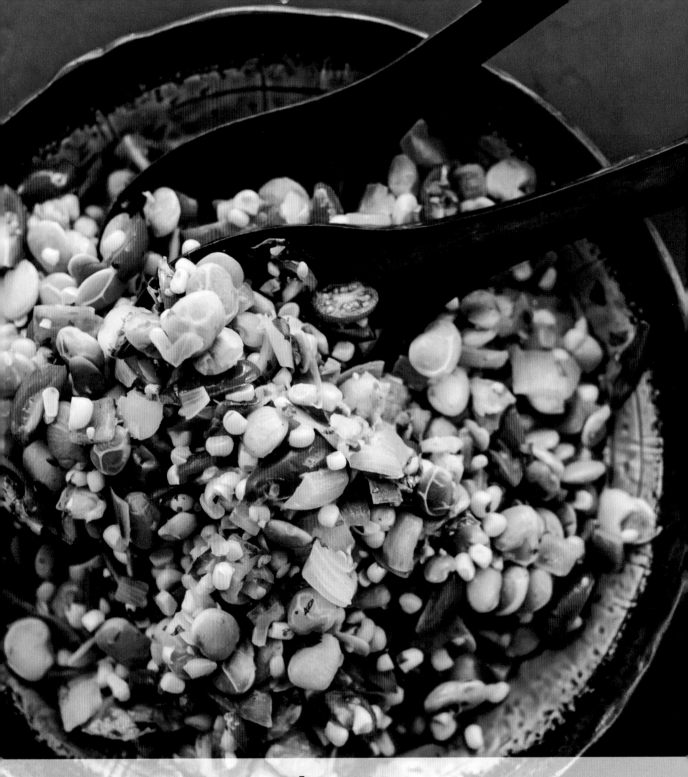

Grape Tomato Succotash, p. 235

Romano Zucchini "Coins"

Makes 1 serving: 1 cup

Easy and amazing can go together. The culinary technique that I call "steam-frying" is what you'll use in this simple side for one; it's basically cooking in a small amount of oil (that's the frying part) in a covered skillet (that's where the steam comes into play) over medium-high heat. The steaming helps you use significantly less oil while creating a luscious result. All that's left to do is to let your taste buds go on a journey to Tuscany.

1. Heat the oil in a large, nonstick skillet over medium-high heat.

2. Working quickly, add the zucchini "coins" in a single layer, sprinkle with the salt and pepper, cover, and cook ("steam-fry") until the bottom of each coin is caramelized, about 3 minutes. Flip each zucchini coin over, cover, and steam-fry until caramelized, about 2 minutes more.

3. Sprinkle with the Romano cheese and basil, and serve.

{ WITH POULTRY, FISH, OR MEAT }

For one serving (full recipe): Slice 3/4 ounce precooked Italian poultry sausage link into thin coins. Heat in a separate nonstick skillet according to package directions. Toss into the skillet with the zucchini at the end of step 2. Skip the Romano. Sprinkle with the basil, and serve.

1 teaspoon extra-virgin olive oil

1 medium zucchini, unpeeled, cut crosswise into 1/3-inch slices ("coins")

1/8 teaspoon sea salt, or to taste

Pinch of freshly ground black pepper, or to taste

1 teaspoon grated Pecorino Romano or Parmigiano-Reggiano cheese

1 teaspoon thinly sliced fresh basil

without

Exchanges/Food Choices: 1 Vegetable, 1 Fat
80 calories, 50 calories from fat, 6g total fat, 1g saturated fat, 0g trans fat, 0mg cholesterol, 330mg sodium, 520mg potassium, 6g total carbohydrate, 2g dietary fiber, 4g sugars, 3g protein, 90mg phosphorus

with

Exchanges/Food Choices: 2 Vegetable, 2 Fat
110 calories, 60 calories from fat, 7g total fat, 1.5g saturated fat, 0g trans fat, 20mg cholesterol, 430mg sodium, 560mg potassium, 7g total carbohydrate, 2g dietary fiber, 4g sugars, 6g protein, 110mg phosphorus

Grilled Artichoke Hearts Provençal

Makes 2 servings: 2 skewers each

2 tablespoons low-sodium vegetable broth
1 tablespoon extra-virgin olive oil
1 large shallot, minced
1 large garlic clove, minced
1 teaspoon fresh lemon juice
2 teaspoons herbes de Provence
1/2 teaspoon sea salt, or to taste
1 (9-ounce) package frozen artichoke hearts, thawed
1 teaspoon lemon zest

Grilled artichoke hearts may not be served at your everyday cookout, but I suggest you change that. These skewers are so flavorful and will add a touch of French flair to a backyard gathering. Multiply the recipe by as many times as you need, and be prepared to have no leftovers. Yes, they're that luscious!

1. Whisk together the broth, oil, shallot, garlic, lemon juice, herbes de Provence, and salt in a medium bowl. Add the artichoke hearts and toss to coat. Let marinate at room temperature for 30–45 minutes, tossing a couple times to assure even marinating.

2. Prepare an outdoor or indoor grill. Insert the artichoke hearts onto 4 reusable or water-soaked bamboo skewers and grill over direct medium-high heat until rich grill marks form, about 4 minutes per side, flipping only once.

3. Sprinkle with the lemon zest, and serve.

{ WITH POULTRY, FISH, OR MEAT }

One serving: Cut 2 ounces boneless, skinless chicken thigh into 6 cubes. Place into a small bowl along with 1/2 teaspoon each extra-virgin olive oil and herbes de Provence. Add a smidgen of sea salt and toss to coat. There's no need for marinating time. Insert onto 1 reusable or water-soaked skewer. Grill next to or after the artichoke hearts until well done, about 4 minutes per side, and serve with 2 artichoke heart skewers.

Full recipe: Cut 4 ounces boneless, skinless chicken thigh into 12 cubes. Place into a small bowl along with 1 teaspoon each extra-virgin olive oil and herbes de Provence. Add a pinch of sea salt and toss to coat. There's no need for marinating time. Insert onto 2 reusable or water-soaked skewers. Grill next to the artichoke hearts until well done, about 4 minutes per side, and serve with the artichoke heart skewers. Alternatively, intersperse the chicken and the artichoke hearts on the same skewers.

without
Exchanges/Food Choices: 3 Vegetable, 1/2 Fat
100 calories, 35 calories from fat, 4g total fat, 0.5g saturated fat, 0g trans fat, 0mg cholesterol, 360mg sodium, 360mg potassium, 16g total carbohydrate, 10g dietary fiber, 2g sugars, 4g protein, 90mg phosphorus

with
Exchanges/Food Choices: 3 Vegetable, 2 Lean Meat, 1/2 Fat
190 calories, 80 calories from fat, 9g total fat, 2g saturated fat, 0g trans fat, 55mg cholesterol, 470mg sodium, 470mg potassium, 16g total carbohydrate, 10g dietary fiber, 2g sugars, 13g protein, 180mg phosphorus

Wok-Sautéed Brussels Sprouts

Makes 4 servings: 3/4 cup each

1 1/4 cups low-sodium vegetable broth

1 1/2 teaspoons brown rice vinegar

1 pound trimmed Brussels sprouts, quartered lengthwise

1 small or 1/2 large red onion, finely diced

1 tablespoon + 1 teaspoon canola or grapeseed oil

1/2 teaspoon sea salt, or to taste

1/4 teaspoon freshly ground black pepper, or to taste

1 teaspoon naturally brewed soy sauce

1 1/2 tablespoons chopped fresh cilantro, or to taste

without
Exchanges/Food Choices: 2 Vegetable, 1 Fat
100 calories, 45 calories from fat, 5g
total fat, 0g saturated fat, 0g trans fat,
0mg cholesterol, 440mg sodium, 420mg
potassium, 12g total carbohydrate, 4g dietary
fiber, 4g sugars, 4g protein, 70mg phosphorus

with
Exchanges/Food Choices: 2 Vegetable, 1 Fat
180 calories, 80 calories from fat,
 9g total fat, 1.5g saturated fat, 0g trans fat,
55mg cholesterol, 470mg sodium,
540mg potassium, 12g total carbohydrate,
4g dietary fiber, 4g sugars, 14g protein,
170mg phosphorus

Brussels sprouts have been a long-celebrated vegetable at Thanksgiving tables in America, but these cute little cabbages are now showing up on family tables all year long. When prepared right, they're a true, savory delight. You'll find this Asian-inspired preparation a unique and delicious way to enjoy this veggie any day.

1. Bring the broth and vinegar to a boil in a wok or extra-large skillet over medium-high heat. Add the Brussels sprouts and onion, and cook while stirring until no liquid remains, about 8 minutes. Add the oil, salt, and pepper, and sauté until the sprouts are crisp-tender and caramelized, about 4 minutes. Sprinkle with the soy sauce and cilantro, and toss to coat. Adjust seasoning.

2. Transfer to individual bowls or a large serving bowl, and serve.

{ WITH POULTRY, FISH, OR MEAT }

One serving: Finely dice 1 1/2 ounces roasted chicken thigh and toss, if desired, with 1/4 teaspoon naturally brewed soy sauce. Then toss with 3/4 cup Brussels sprouts mixture.

Full recipe: Finely dice 6 ounces roasted chicken thigh and toss, if desired, with 1 teaspoon naturally brewed soy sauce. Stir chicken into the skillet after the Brussels sprouts are lightly caramelized and sauté for 1 minute more; sprinkle with the soy sauce and cilantro in the main recipe.

Collard Greens in Sweet Onion Broth

Makes 4 servings: about 1 cup each

You'll get a real kick in the palate out of this southern-style side dish. These savory, slow-simmered collard greens have a peppery bite that's deliciously balanced with a just-right amount of sweet onion broth. It's comforting.

1. Heat the oil in a Dutch oven over medium heat. Add the onion and lemon juice, and sauté until the onion is softened, about 8 minutes. Add the garlic and sauté until fragrant, about 1 minute.

2. Add the broth, collard greens, black pepper, salt, and hot pepper flakes, and bring to a boil over high heat. Cover, reduce heat to medium-low, and simmer until the collard greens are tender, about 50 minutes. (Note: Cooking time will vary.) Adjust seasoning.

3. Transfer the collard greens with broth to individual serving bowls. Serve with the lemon wedges on the side.

{ WITH POULTRY, FISH, OR MEAT }

One serving: Dice 3/4 ounce lean, uncured ham or Canadian bacon. Heat in a nonstick skillet over medium-high heat until lightly browned, about 1 1/2 minutes. Stir into one of the servings in step 3.

Full recipe: Dice 3 ounces lean, uncured ham or Canadian bacon. Stir into the collard greens after they've been simmering for 40 minutes in step 2.

1 tablespoon extra-virgin olive oil

1 large sweet onion, diced

1 teaspoon fresh lemon juice

4 large garlic cloves, thinly sliced

1 1/3 cups low-sodium vegetable broth

1 pound collard greens, stems and thick ribs removed, leaves cut into 1-inch-wide strips

3/4 teaspoon freshly ground black pepper, or to taste

1/2 teaspoon sea salt, or to taste

1/4 teaspoon dried hot pepper flakes, or to taste

4 lemon wedges

without

Exchanges/Food Choices: 2 Vegetable, 1/2 Fat
90 calories, 35 calories from fat, 4g total fat, 0.5g saturated fat, 0g trans fat, 0mg cholesterol, 360mg sodium, 210mg potassium, 13g total carbohydrate, 4g dietary fiber, 5g sugars, 3g protein, 50mg phosphorus

with

Exchanges/Food Choices: 2 Vegetable, 1 Lean Meat, 1 Fat
120 calories, 40 calories from fat, 4.5g total fat, 0.5g saturated fat, 0g trans fat, 15mg cholesterol, 480mg sodium, 270mg potassium, 13g total carbohydrate, 4g dietary fiber, 5g sugars, 7g protein, 90mg phosphorus

Garlic Sautéed Rapini with Tart Cherries

Makes 4 servings: about 1 cup each

1 whole small garlic bulb

1 tablespoon extra-virgin olive oil, divided

1/2 cup low-sodium vegetable broth

3 tablespoons dried tart cherries

1 (1-pound) bunch rapini (broccoli raab), stems trimmed

1/4 teaspoon sea salt, or to taste

1/4 teaspoon freshly ground black pepper, or to taste

1/4 teaspoon dried hot pepper flakes

1 tablespoon red wine vinegar

Try this taste-bud thriller. It's got sweet, salty, and bitter, plus a hint of heat, to please anyone into big taste. The rapini's noteworthy bitterness is beautifully balanced in this side dish preparation with pleasant pops of cherries.

1. Cut the top portion off of the garlic to expose all the cloves. Rub with 1/2 teaspoon oil. Wrap in recycled aluminum foil. Bake in a toaster oven (or preheat conventional oven) at 375°F until fully softened, about 25 minutes. When cool enough to handle, squeeze the softened garlic cloves from the skins. Fully smash the cloves.

2. Bring the broth, cherries, and garlic to a boil in a large, deep skillet over medium-high heat. Add the rapini and cook while tossing until no liquid remains, about 3 minutes.

3. Add the remaining 2 1/2 teaspoons oil, salt, black pepper, and hot pepper flakes, and toss with tongs until the rapini is crisp-tender, about 3 minutes. Toss with the vinegar. Adjust seasoning.

4. Transfer the rapini to individual plates or a platter, and serve.

{ WITH POULTRY, FISH, OR MEAT }

One serving: Thinly slice 3/4 ounce precooked sweet Italian poultry sausage link into half moons. Heat in a nonstick skillet according to package directions. Toss into one of the servings of rapini when ready to serve.

Full recipe: Thinly slice a 3-ounce precooked sweet Italian poultry sausage link into half moons. Add to the skillet in step 3 after adding the oil, salt, black pepper, and hot pepper flakes.

without
Exchanges/Food Choices: 1/2 Fruit, 1 Vegetable, 1 Fat
90 calories, 35 calories from fat, 4g total fat, 0.5g saturated fat, 0g trans fat, 0mg cholesterol, 200mg sodium, 280mg potassium, 11g total carbohydrate, 3g dietary fiber, 5g sugars, 4g protein, 90mg phosphorus

with
Exchanges/Food Choices: 1/2 Fruit, 1 Vegetable, 1/2 Medium-Fat Meat, 1 Fat
130 calories, 60 calories from fat, 7g total fat, 1.5g saturated fat, 0g trans fat, 20mg cholesterol, 370mg sodium, 320mg potassium, 12g total carbohydrate, 3g dietary fiber, 5g sugars, 7g protein, 130mg phosphorus

Citrus Braised Kale

Makes 4 servings: 1 1/4 cups each

1 teaspoon unsalted butter or
   extra-virgin olive oil

1 pound chopped fresh kale

1/4 cup freshly squeezed orange juice
   + 1 teaspoon orange zest

1/4 teaspoon + 1/8 teaspoon sea salt,
   or to taste

1/4 teaspoon freshly ground black
   pepper, or to taste

1/8 teaspoon dried hot pepper flakes,
   or to taste

Kale is a popular green for a good reason. It's super nutrient rich and packs a punch of delightful yet slightly bitter tones. In this recipe, its taste is totally balanced by the fresh sweetness from the orange, richness from the hint of butter, and "heat" from the hot pepper flakes. To top that, it's simple to prepare. So make this kale recipe a go-to side often.

1. Melt the butter in a Dutch oven over medium-high heat. Add the kale and sauté by tossing with tongs until just wilted, about 5 minutes.

2. Add the orange juice, salt, black pepper, and hot pepper flakes, and toss to combine. Cover, reduce heat to medium-low, and cook until fully softened, about 5 minutes, stirring once during braising. Adjust seasoning.

3. Sprinkle with the orange zest, and serve.

{ WITH POULTRY, FISH, OR MEAT }

One serving: Finely chop 1 slice of crisp-cooked, hardwood-smoked, uncured turkey bacon or Sunday bacon and toss onto one serving of the kale at serving time.

Full recipe: Finely chop 4 slices of crisp-cooked, hardwood-smoked, uncured turkey bacon or Sunday bacon and toss into the kale before adjusting the seasoning in step 2.

without
Exchanges/Food Choices: 2 Vegetable, 1/2 Fat
70 calories, 20 calories from fat, 2g total fat, 0.5g saturated fat, 0g trans fat, 5mg cholesterol, 260mg sodium, 590mg potassium, 12g total carbohydrate, 2g dietary fiber, 1g sugars, 5g protein, 110mg phosphorus

with
Exchanges/Food Choices: 2 Vegetable, 1 Lean Meat, 1/2 Fat
110 calories, 30 calories from fat, 3.5g total fat, 0.5g saturated fat, 0g trans fat, 30mg cholesterol, 460mg sodium, 660mg potassium, 12g total carbohydrate, 2g dietary fiber, 1g sugars, 11g protein, 160mg phosphorus

Rosemary Carrot and Cabbage Sauté

Makes 4 servings: 1 rounded cup each

Cabbage becomes a fully satisfying side with this sautéed preparation, fragranced with fresh rosemary and accented with caramelized onions and carrots. The generous splash of apple cider vinegar marries it all together. It's a surprising taste-bud pleaser.

1. Heat 1 tablespoon oil in a wok or nonstick Dutch oven over medium-high heat. Add the onion, carrots, 1 tablespoon vinegar, and 1/4 teaspoon salt, and sauté until the onion is softened and begins to caramelize, about 5 minutes. Add the cabbage and sauté until the cabbage is nearly wilted and carrots are crisp-tender, about 8 minutes. Stir in the rosemary, pepper, and the remaining 1 tablespoon vinegar, 1 teaspoon oil, and 1/2 teaspoon salt, and continue to sauté until the cabbage is wilted as desired, about 2 minutes. Adjust seasoning.

2. Transfer to a large serving bowl or individual bowls, and serve immediately.

{ WITH POULTRY, FISH, OR MEAT }

One serving: Finely dice 1/2 ounce lean, uncured Canadian bacon. Heat in a nonstick skillet over medium-high heat until lightly browned, about 1 1/2 minutes. Transfer 1 rounded cup carrot-cabbage mixture to a small serving bowl and stir in the Canadian bacon. Use 1/2 teaspoon instead of 3/4 teaspoon sea salt in the main recipe, and adjust seasoning as needed.

Full recipe: Finely dice 2 ounces lean, uncured Canadian bacon. Heat in a nonstick skillet over medium-high heat until lightly browned, about 1 1/2 minutes. Stir into the carrot-cabbage mixture in step 1 before adjusting seasoning. Use 1/2 teaspoon instead of 3/4 teaspoon sea salt in the main recipe.

1 tablespoon + 1 teaspoon extra-virgin olive oil

1 jumbo yellow onion, halved, very thinly sliced

1 cup small baby carrots, quartered lengthwise

2 tablespoons apple cider vinegar, divided

3/4 teaspoon sea salt, divided

1/2 head green cabbage, cored, thinly sliced (7 cups sliced)

1 teaspoon finely chopped fresh rosemary, or to taste

1/2 teaspoon freshly ground black pepper, or to taste

without
Exchanges/Food Choices: 3 Vegetable, 1 Fat
110 calories, 40 calories from fat, 5g total fat, 0.5g saturated fat, 0g trans fat, 0mg cholesterol, 480mg sodium, 310mg potassium, 17g total carbohydrate, 5g dietary fiber, 8g sugars, 3g protein, 50mg phosphorus

with
Exchanges/Food Choices: 3 Vegetable, 1/2 Lean Meat, 1 Fat
130 calories, 50 calories from fat, 6g total fat, 1g saturated fat, 0g trans fat, 5mg cholesterol, 470mg sodium, 350mg potassium, 17g total carbohydrate, 5g dietary fiber, 8g sugars, 5g protein, 80mg phosphorus

Purée of Cauliflower

Makes 4 servings: about 3/4 cup each

1 medium head cauliflower, cut into small florets (6 cups florets;)

1/3 cup plain unsweetened almond milk or other plant-based milk

1 tablespoon + 1 teaspoon extra-virgin olive oil

1 large garlic clove, minced

1/4 teaspoon + 1/8 teaspoon sea salt, or to taste

1 teaspoon unsalted butter, cut into 4 pats

1 tablespoon minced fresh chives or scallion

without
Exchanges/Food Choices: 1 Vegetable, 1 Fat
90 calories, 60 calories from fat, 6g total fat, 1.5g saturated fat, 0g trans fat, 5mg cholesterol, 250mg sodium, 220mg potassium, 7g total carbohydrate, 3g dietary fiber, 3g sugars, 3g protein, 50mg phosphorus

with
Exchanges/Food Choices: 2 Vegetable, 1 1/2 Fat
120 calories, 70 calories from fat, 8g total fat, 1g saturated fat, 0g trans fat, 5mg cholesterol, 450mg sodium, 530mg potassium, 10g total carbohydrate, 4g dietary fiber, 5g sugars, 6g protein, 140mg phosphorus

There's an intriguing twist to this side. Instead of mashing potatoes, you'll be whipping up cauliflower and serving it just like mashed potatoes. You can drizzle your serving with gravy, if you like. It's deliciously comforting in a calorie-conscious way.

1. Bring a large saucepan of water to a boil over high heat. Add the cauliflower and boil until very tender, about 12 minutes.

2. Meanwhile, whisk together the almond milk, oil, garlic, and salt in a small saucepan, and keep hot over low heat.

3. Drain the cauliflower and add to a food processor. Add the almond milk mixture, cover, and purée until smooth. Adjust seasoning.

4. Transfer to individual bowls, top each with a butter pat, sprinkle with the chives, and serve.

{ WITH POULTRY, FISH, OR MEAT }

One serving: Drain excess liquids from 1/3 rounded cup of the "With Poultry, Fish, or Meat" version of Saucy Mushrooms (page 216). Serve the mushrooms on top of 3/4 cup whipped cauliflower before sprinkling with the chives in step 4. Skip the butter.

Full recipe: Drain excess liquids from about 1 1/2 cups of the "With Poultry, Fish, or Meat" version of Saucy Mushrooms (page 216). Serve the mushrooms on top of the whipped cauliflower before sprinkling with the chives in step 4. Skip the butter.

Veggie Fried Rice

Makes 4 servings: 1/2 rounded cup each

This isn't your typical fried rice because it isn't laden with grease. Luckily, it's still loaded with Asian taste and sensory appeal. Enjoy it with chopsticks to add worldly flair and to help you savor this colorful side slowly.

1. Heat the oil in a wok over medium-high heat. Add the bell pepper, garlic, Serrano pepper, and the white part of the scallions, and stir-fry until the scallions begin to caramelize, about 2 minutes.

2. Add the chilled rice, mushrooms, and ginger, and stir-fry until the rice mixture is browned, about 6 minutes. Add the soy sauce, cilantro, and the green part of the scallions, and stir to combine.

3. Sprinkle with the sesame seeds, and serve.

{ WITH POULTRY, FISH, OR MEAT }

One serving: Finely dice 1 1/2 ounces pork tenderloin, toss with 1/2 teaspoon toasted sesame oil and 1/4 teaspoon naturally brewed soy sauce, and sauté in a small, nonstick skillet over medium-high heat until done, about 2 minutes. Stir into 1/2 rounded cup fried rice before sprinkling with the sesame seeds in step 3.

Full recipe: Finely dice 6 ounces pork tenderloin, toss with 2 teaspoons toasted sesame oil and 1 teaspoon naturally brewed soy sauce, and add to the wok along with the rice in step 2.

---

2 tablespoons canola or peanut oil

1 large red bell pepper, finely diced

2 large garlic cloves, minced

1 Serrano pepper, with some seeds, minced

3 scallions, thinly sliced, green and white parts separated

1 3/4 cups cooked long-grain brown rice, chilled

1 cup thinly sliced fresh shiitake mushrooms with stems removed

1 1/2 teaspoons freshly grated gingerroot

1 1/2 tablespoons naturally brewed soy sauce, or to taste

3 tablespoons chopped fresh cilantro

1 teaspoon black or white sesame seeds, toasted

with
Exchanges/Food Choices: 1 Starch, 1 Vegetable, 1 Fat
170 calories, 70 calories from fat, 8g total fat, 0.5g saturated fat, 0g trans fat, 0mg cholesterol, 360mg sodium, 240mg potassium, 21g total carbohydrate, 3g dietary fiber, 3g sugars, 4g protein, 100mg phosphorus

with
Exchanges/Food Choices: 1 Starch, 1 Vegetable, 1 Lean Meat, 2 Fat
240 calories, 100 calories from fat, 12g total fat, 1.5g saturated fat, 0g trans fat, 20mg cholesterol, 450mg sodium, 370mg potassium, 21g total carbohydrate, 3g dietary fiber, 3g sugars, 12g protein, 180mg phosphorus

Tahini-Dressed Roasted Eggplant

1 large (1 1/4-pound) eggplant, cut crosswise into 12 slices

Olive oil cooking spray

1/4 teaspoon + 1/8 teaspoon sea salt, or to taste

3 tablespoons tahini

3 tablespoons unsweetened green tea or vegetable broth

Juice of 1 small lemon (2 tablespoons)

1/2 tablespoon extra-virgin olive oil

1 large garlic clove, minced

Pinch ground cumin, or to taste

16 large fresh flat-leaf parsley leaves + 4 fresh flat-leaf parsley sprigs

Like Middle Eastern cuisine? You'll love this dazzling side dish of tahini-dressed roasted eggplant rounds, arranged in layers that are lovingly interspersed with fresh parsley. It's a show-stopper, so also consider serving it as a stand-alone appetizer. Hint: If you have leftovers, add the eggplant and tahini dressing to a food processor and purée with an extra splash of lemon juice to make roasted eggplant dip.

1. Preheat the oven to 450°F. Spritz both sides of the eggplant slices with olive oil cooking spray. Sprinkle with 1/4 teaspoon salt. Arrange onto a large, unbleached parchment paper–lined baking sheet. Roast in the oven until fully cooked and lightly browned, about 30 minutes, flipping over eggplant rounds about halfway through the roasting process.

2. Meanwhile, whisk together until smooth the tahini, tea, lemon juice, oil, garlic, cumin, and the remaining 1/8 teaspoon salt in a medium bowl or liquid measuring cup. Adjust seasoning.

3. Onto 4 plates or a platter, arrange stacks of 3 eggplant rounds, placing the largest round on the bottom of each stack. Alternatively, fan out the eggplant rounds on a plate rather than stacking them. Position the parsley leaves between the layers, allowing the leaves to peek out. Drizzle with tahini dressing, garnish with the parsley sprigs, and serve warm or at room temperature.

{ WITH POULTRY, FISH, OR MEAT }

One serving: Combine 2 ounces extra-lean, ground, grass-fed beef or lamb with 1 tablespoon each plain fat-free Greek yogurt and grated yellow onion, 1/2 teaspoon finely chopped fresh mint, and a pinch each of sea salt and freshly ground black pepper. Form into a thin (4-inch diameter) patty. Prepare in a small, nonstick skillet over medium-high heat until done, about 2 1/2 minutes per side, gently flipping over once during the cooking process. Serve one of the eggplant stacks on top of the beef patty or fan the 3 eggplant rounds around the patty. Alternatively, serve the beef patty in place of the center eggplant round—sort of like a hamburger, where the eggplant rounds act somewhat like the bun.

Full recipe: Combine 8 ounces extra-lean, ground, grass-fed beef or lamb with 1/4 cup each plain fat-free Greek yogurt and grated yellow onion, 2 teaspoons finely chopped fresh mint, and 1/4 teaspoon each sea salt and freshly ground black pepper. Form into 4 thin (4-inch diameter) patties. Prepare in a large, nonstick skillet (in batches) over medium-high heat until done, about 2 1/2 minutes per side, gently flipping over once during the cooking process. Serve each of the eggplant stacks on top of a beef patty or fan eggplant rounds around the patties. Alternatively, serve a beef patty in place of each center eggplant round—sort of like hamburgers, where the eggplant rounds act somewhat like the buns.

without
Exchanges/Food Choices: 2 Vegetable, 1 1/2 Fat
120 calories, 70 calories from fat, 8g total fat,
1g saturated fat, 0g trans fat, 0mg cholesterol,
220mg sodium, 210mg potassium, 13g total
carbohydrate, 3g dietary fiber, 4g sugars,
3g protein, 110mg phosphorus

with
Exchanges/Food Choices: 2 Vegetable,
2 Lean Meat, 2 Fat
200 calories, 100 calories from fat, 11g total fat,
2.5g saturated fat, 0g trans fat, 30mg cholesterol,
400mg sodium, 390mg potassium, 15g total
carbohydrate, 4g dietary fiber, 5g sugars,
15g protein, 220mg phosphorus

Spaghetti Squash a Cacio e Pepe

Makes 4 servings: 1 rounded cup each

1 (3 1/2-pound) spaghetti squash, halved lengthwise, seeds and stringy pulp removed

Olive oil cooking spray

1/2 teaspoon minced fresh rosemary

2 teaspoons whole black peppercorns

3 tablespoons finely grated Pecorino Romano or Parmigiano-Reggiano cheese

1/4 teaspoon sea salt, or to taste

I often enjoy the traditional version of this recipe using regular spaghetti, but this roasted spaghetti squash version provides an interesting taste, texture, and nutritional twist. The toasted peppercorns create so much pow. In fact, the pepper is the key ingredient in this Roman-inspired recipe.

1. Preheat the oven to 350°F. In a large baking dish lined with unbleached parchment paper, place the spaghetti squash halves cut side up, spritz with olive oil cooking spray, and sprinkle with the rosemary. Turn the squash halves over, cover the entire baking dish with foil, and roast until the squash is fork-tender, about 1 hour 10 minutes. (Note: Roasting time varies based on size of squash.)

2. Meanwhile, toast the peppercorns in a small skillet over medium-high heat until fragrant and peppercorns begin to "pop," about 2 1/2–3 minutes. Coarsely crush the peppercorns using a mortar and pestle or by pulsing a few times in a coffee grinder.

3. Let the squash stand, uncovered, until just cool enough to handle. Scrape the flesh out of the skins into spaghetti-like strands. Add the cheese, salt, and half of the pepper, and toss quickly using tongs. Divide among 4 salad plates or bowls, sprinkle with the remaining pepper, and serve immediately.

WITH POULTRY, FISH, OR MEAT

One serving: Simmer two (3/4-ounce) fully cooked poultry Italian meatballs in 1/3 cup marinara sauce of choice (page 191) in a small saucepan until the meatballs are fully reheated. Cut meatballs in half. Transfer 1 rounded cup spaghetti squash in step 3 to a serving bowl. Do not add the cheese or salt, but add the pepper as instructed. Ladle the meatballs and sauce onto the serving. Garnish with a fresh basil sprig, if desired, and serve as an entrée instead of a side.

Full recipe: Simmer eight (3/4-ounce) fully cooked poultry Italian meatballs in 1 1/3 cups marinara sauce of choice (page 191) in a large saucepan until the meatballs are fully reheated. Cut meatballs in half. In step 3, do not add the cheese and salt, but add the pepper as instructed. Just before serving, ladle the meatballs and sauce onto the spaghetti squash. Garnish with fresh basil sprigs, if desired, and serve as an entrée instead of a side.

without
Exchanges/Food Choices: 4 Vegetable, 1/2 Fat
110 calories, 25 calories from fat, 3g total fat,
1g saturated fat, 0g trans fat, 5mg cholesterol,
320mg sodium, 310mg potassium, 20g total
carbohydrate, 4g dietary fiber, 8g sugars,
3g protein, 60mg phosphorus

with
Exchanges/Food Choices: 5 Vegetable,
1 Medium-Fat Meat, 1/2 Fat
220 calories, 90 calories from fat, 10g total fat,
2.5g saturated fat, 0g trans fat, 55mg cholesterol,
600mg sodium, 630mg potassium, 26g total
carbohydrate, 6g dietary fiber, 12g sugars,
11g protein, 160mg phosphorus

Sticky Thai Quinoa

1 tablespoon canola or peanut oil

1 sweet onion, finely chopped

1 tablespoon freshly grated
   lemongrass

Juice of 1/2 lime (1 tablespoon)

3/4 teaspoon sea salt, divided

2 teaspoons freshly grated gingerroot

1/4 teaspoon ground turmeric

1 cup quinoa, rinsed and well drained

1 7/8 cups low-sodium vegetable
   broth

3 tablespoons light coconut milk

1/4 cup thinly sliced fresh basil
   + 6 fresh basil sprigs

You may have had or at least heard of sticky rice, but have you had sticky quinoa? Now is your chance. But don't prepare this recipe just because it's sticky; make it because it's sumptuous. The culinary synergy of lemongrass, ginger, and coconut milk provides Thai flair and fragrance, and the turmeric imparts a distinguishing yellow hue. It's lovely.

1. Heat the oil in a large saucepan over medium heat. Add the onion, lemongrass, lime juice, and 1/4 teaspoon salt, and sauté until the onion is fully softened, about 8 minutes. Add the ginger and turmeric, and sauté for 1 minute.

2. Add the quinoa, broth, and the remaining 1/2 teaspoon salt, and bring to a boil over high heat. Cover, reduce heat to low, and cook until the quinoa is al dente and the broth is absorbed, about 20 minutes, only partially covering during the final 5 minutes. Immediately stir in the coconut milk. Adjust seasoning.

3. Stir in the sliced basil, garnish with the basil sprigs, and serve.

{ WITH POULTRY, FISH, OR MEAT }

One serving: Cut 2 ounces turkey tenderloin into 8 cubes, or use 8 shrimp. Insert onto a reusable or water-soaked bamboo skewer. Spritz the turkey with cooking spray and season with 1/8 teaspoon curry powder and a pinch of sea salt. Grill or pan-grill over direct medium-high heat until well done, about 4 minutes per side. Serve the skewer on 2/3 cup quinoa.

Full recipe: Cut 12 ounces turkey tenderloin into 48 cubes, or use 48 shrimp. Insert onto 6 reusable or water-soaked bamboo skewers. Spritz the turkey with cooking spray and season with 3/4 teaspoon curry powder and 1/4 teaspoon sea salt. Grill or pan-grill over direct medium-high heat until well done, about 4 minutes per side. Serve the skewers on the quinoa.

without
Exchanges/Food Choices: 1 1/2 Starch, 1 Fat
150 calories, 40 calories from fat, 4.5g total fat,
0.5g saturated fat, 0g trans fat, 0mg cholesterol,
340mg sodium, 240mg potassium, 24g total
carbohydrate, 3g dietary fiber, 5g sugars,
5g protein, 150mg phosphorus

with
Exchanges/Food Choices: 1 1/2 Starch,
2 Lean Meat
220 calories, 50 calories from fat, 5g total fat,
1g saturated fat, 0g trans fat, 35mg cholesterol,
460mg sodium, 380mg potassium, 24g total
carbohydrate, 3g dietary fiber, 5g sugars,
18g protein, 250mg phosphorus

Citrus Mint Farro with Almonds

Makes 10 servings: 1/2 cup each

1 1/2 tablespoons extra-virgin olive oil

1 medium red onion, diced

Juice of 1/2 lemon (1 1/2 tablespoons)

1 1/4 teaspoons sea salt, divided

1 3/4 cups whole farro, rinsed and drained

2 1/2 cups low-sodium vegetable broth

Juice of 1 large dark red or pink grapefruit (1 cup)

3 tablespoons finely chopped fresh mint

1/2 teaspoon freshly ground black pepper, or to taste

3/4 cup sliced natural almonds, toasted

without
Exchanges/Food Choices: 2 Starch, 1 Fat
180 calories, 60 calories from fat, 6g total fat, 0.5g saturated fat, 0g trans fat, 0mg cholesterol, 330mg sodium, 210mg potassium, 28g total carbohydrate, 4g dietary fiber, 3g sugars, 5g protein, 150mg phosphorus

with
Exchanges/Food Choices: 2 Starch, 1 Lean Meat, 1 1/2 Fat
240 calories, 90 calories from fat, 10g total fat, 1.5g saturated fat, 0g trans fat, 35mg cholesterol, 420mg sodium, 290mg potassium, 28g total carbohydrate, 4g dietary fiber, 3g sugars, 12g protein, 210mg phosphorus

Farro is a whole grain that's full of chewiness and nuttiness. A petite serving provides great satisfaction. When simmered in a citrusy broth, finished with fresh mint, and topped with toasty almonds, it's pure happiness in a bowl.

1. Heat the oil in a large saucepan over medium-high heat. Add the onion, lemon juice, and 1/4 teaspoon salt, and sauté until the onion is softened and lightly caramelized, about 6 minutes.

2. Add the farro, broth, grapefruit juice, and the remaining 1 teaspoon salt, and bring to a boil over high heat. Reduce the heat to low, cover, and simmer until the farro is desired tenderness, about 40 minutes.

3. Stir in the mint and pepper. Adjust seasoning.

4. Transfer to a serving bowl or individual bowls, sprinkle with the almonds, and serve warm.

{ WITH POULTRY, FISH, OR MEAT }

One serving: Season 1 ounce rotisserie chicken thigh meat with about 1/8 teaspoon freshly ground black pepper. Transfer 1/2 cup farro to a small serving bowl before adjusting seasoning in step 3. Immediately stir the chicken into the farro, and serve with almonds on top.

Full recipe: Season 10 ounces rotisserie chicken dark meat with 1 teaspoon freshly ground black pepper. Stir into the farro along with the mint in step 3.

Grape Tomato Succotash

Makes 4 servings: 1 rounded cup each

Succotash is usually associated with summertime cuisine, when corn is in season. But this recipe is designed to be enjoyed anytime you're able to pick up a pint of grape tomatoes. Since you can use frozen lima beans and corn here, you can savor this veggie dish often. It's as colorful as it is flavorful.

1. Heat the oil in a large skillet over medium-high heat. Add the onion, lima beans, corn, and jalapeño, and sauté until the vegetables are heated through, about 3 minutes. Add the sunflower milk beverage and salt, and sauté until the vegetables are tender and liquid is fully reduced, about 6 minutes. Add the tomatoes and vinegar, and sauté until the tomatoes are heated through, about 1 minute. Stir in the cilantro. Adjust seasoning.

2. Transfer to a serving bowl or individual bowls, garnish with additional cilantro, if desired, and serve.

WITH POULTRY, FISH, OR MEAT

One serving: Use a pinch less sea salt than in the main recipe. Cut 1 slice hickory-smoked, uncured bacon crosswise into 1/3-inch-wide slices. Sauté the bacon in a small skillet over medium heat until fully browned and crisp, about 8 minutes. Transfer the bacon with a slotted spoon to unbleached paper towels to drain. After stirring in the cilantro in step 1, transfer 1 rounded cup succotash to a small serving bowl. Sprinkle with the bacon.

Full recipe: Use 1/4 teaspoon sea salt in the main recipe instead of 1/2 teaspoon. Cut 4 slices hickory-smoked, uncured bacon crosswise into 1/3-inch-wide slices. Sauté the bacon in a large skillet over medium heat until browned and crisp, about 8 minutes. Transfer the bacon with a slotted spoon to unbleached paper towels to drain. After stirring in the cilantro in step 1, stir in the bacon.

2 teaspoons extra-virgin olive oil

1 medium red onion, diced

1 pound fresh lima beans in pods, shelled, or 10 ounces thawed frozen lima beans (2 cups)

1 cup fresh (from 2 medium ears) or thawed frozen yellow sweet corn

1/2 small jalapeño pepper, with seeds, thinly sliced crosswise

3/4 cup plain unsweetened sunflower milk beverage or almond milk

1/2 teaspoon sea salt

1 pint grape tomatoes, quartered lengthwise

1 tablespoon apple cider vinegar

3 tablespoons finely chopped fresh cilantro

without
Exchanges/Food Choices: 1 Starch, 1 Vegetable, 1 Fat
160 calories, 35 calories from fat, 4g total fat, 0.5g saturated fat, 0g trans fat, 0mg cholesterol, 360mg sodium, 640mg potassium, 28g total carbohydrate, 6g dietary fiber, 5g sugars, 7g protein, 220mg phosphorus

with
Exchanges/Food Choices: 1 Starch, 1 1/2 Vegetable, 1 Medium-Fat Meat
190 calories, 60 calories from fat, 6g total fat, 1.5g saturated fat, 0g trans fat, 5mg cholesterol, 360mg sodium, 670mg potassium, 28g total carbohydrate, 6g dietary fiber, 5g sugars, 9g protein, 250mg phosphorus

White Beans Caliente

Makes 4 servings: 1/2 cup each

2 teaspoons unrefined peanut oil or canola oil

1 (15-ounce) can Great Northern or cannellini beans, gently rinsed and drained (1 1/2 cups)

3/4 cup spicy pico de gallo

1/2 teaspoon finely chopped fresh oregano

1/8 teaspoon ground cumin, or to taste

without
Exchanges/Food Choices: 1 Starch, 1/2 Vegetable, 1/2 Fat
120 calories, 20 calories from fat, 2.5g total fat, 0g saturated fat, 0g trans fat, 0mg cholesterol, 340mg sodium, 330mg potassium, 20g total carbohydrate, 5g dietary fiber, 5g sugars, 6g protein, 120mg phosphorus

with
Exchanges/Food Choices: 1 Starch, 1/2 Vegetable, 1 Lean Meat, 1 Fat
190 calories, 50 calories from fat, 6g total fat, 1.5g saturated fat, 0g trans fat, 55mg cholesterol, 450mg sodium, 440mg potassium, 20g total carbohydrate, 5g dietary fiber, 5g sugars, 15g protein, 210mg phosphorus

This zippy side with its Mexican flair is fast to fix and will fill you up. It's a perfect protein-rich pairing for a vegetarian entrée that's not so protein rich. It's versatile, too. Try it as the main ingredient in a burrito. If you have leftovers, serve chilled as a bean salad with a squirt of lime.

1. Heat the oil in a small saucepan over medium-high heat. Add the beans, pico de gallo, oregano, and cumin. Cook while stirring until the beans are fully heated and no excess liquid remains, about 6 minutes.

2. Transfer to individual bowls or a medium serving bowl, and serve hot or at room temperature.

WITH POULTRY, FISH, OR MEAT

One serving: Spritz 2 ounces (1/2 of a 4-ounce) boneless, skinless chicken thigh with cooking spray, season with a smidgen each of sea salt and chili powder, and grill over medium-high heat until done, about 4 minutes per side. Finely dice, and stir into 1/2 cup bean mixture when serving in step 2.

Full recipe: Spritz 2 (4-ounce) boneless, skinless chicken thighs with cooking spray, season with 1/8 teaspoon each sea salt and chili powder, and grill over medium-high heat until done, about 5 minutes per side. Finely dice and stir into the bean mixture in the saucepan at the end of step 1.

Szechuan Edamame

Makes 4 servings: 3/4 cup each

Edamame is often enjoyed straight from the pod, sprinkled with salt. Simple is good, but edamame is so much more versatile than you might realize. Consider going for a bit of intrigue from time to time. Here's the way I recommend doing it: ...nice and spicy with a hint of citrus.

1. Prepare the edamame according to package directions. Drain well.

2. Heat the oil in a wok or large skillet over medium heat. Add the edamame, ginger, and hot pepper flakes, increase heat to high, and stir-fry until the edamame begins to caramelize, about 2 1/2 minutes. Add the soy sauce, garlic, salt, and 1 teaspoon orange zest, and stir-fry for 30 seconds. Adjust seasoning.

3. Transfer to a medium bowl or individual bowls, garnish with the remaining 1/2 teaspoon orange zest, and serve.

WITH POULTRY, FISH, OR MEAT

One serving: Pan-grill a 3/4-ounce portion of beef tenderloin or sirloin over medium-high heat until medium-rare or medium, about 1 1/2 minutes per side. Finely dice, sprinkle with a smidgen of sea salt, and toss into 3/4 cup edamame when serving in step 3.

Full recipe: Finely dice 3 ounces uncooked beef tenderloin or sirloin, sprinkle with 1/8 teaspoon sea salt, and add along with the edamame, ginger, and hot pepper flakes in step 2.

1 pound frozen shelled edamame (3 1/2 cups)

2 teaspoons toasted sesame oil

2 teaspoons freshly grated gingerroot

1/4 teaspoon dried hot pepper flakes

1 1/2 teaspoons naturally brewed soy sauce

1 large garlic clove, minced

1/4 teaspoon sea salt, or to taste

1 1/2 teaspoons orange zest, divided

without
Exchanges/Food Choices: 1 Starch, 2 Lean Meat
160 calories, 70 calories from fat, 8g total fat, 1g saturated fat, 0g trans fat, 0mg cholesterol, 270mg sodium, 510mg potassium, 12g total carbohydrate, 6g dietary fiber, 3g sugars, 13g protein, 190mg phosphorus

with
Exchanges/Food Choices: 1 Starch, 2 Lean Meat, 1 Fat
190 calories, 80 calories from fat, 10g total fat, 1.5g saturated fat, 0g trans fat, 10mg cholesterol, 350mg sodium, 560mg potassium, 12g total carbohydrate, 6g dietary fiber, 3g sugars, 17g protein, 230mg phosphorus

Tuscan Skillet Red Beans

Makes 4 servings: 3/4 cup each

2 1/2 teaspoons extra-virgin olive oil

1 medium yellow onion, finely diced

1/2 cup finely diced fennel + 1 tablespoon chopped fennel fronds

3 cups packed chopped fresh kale leaves (3 ounces)

2 large garlic cloves, thinly sliced

1 1/2 tablespoons red wine vinegar

1/2 teaspoon sea salt, divided

1/2 cup low-sodium vegetable broth

1 (15-ounce) can no-salt-added red kidney beans, drained (1 1/2 cups)

1 teaspoon lemon zest

You may think the greatest part of this side is how it's served . . . directly from the skillet. Then once you take a bite, you'll realize it's the great taste that makes this a winning dish. It has distinctive Italian flavor along with so much color and texture appeal. The red beans provide a different twist, since white beans are more traditional. Also consider using one or more varieties of cooked heirloom Italian beans, such as Borlotti, Pavoni, or Zolfini beans.

1. Heat the oil in a large, nonstick skillet over medium-high heat. Add the onion, the diced fennel, kale, garlic, vinegar, and 1/4 teaspoon salt, and sauté until the onion is fully softened and begins to caramelize and the kale is wilted, about 8 minutes.

2. Add the broth, beans, fennel fronds, and the remaining 1/4 teaspoon salt, and sauté until the liquid is fully reduced, about 3 minutes. Adjust seasoning.

3. Sprinkle with the lemon zest, and enjoy warm served from the skillet.

{ WITH POULTRY, FISH, OR MEAT }

One serving: Heat 2 (3/4-ounce) fully cooked poultry Italian meatballs according to package directions, cut into 3 slices each, nestle on top of one of the servings, and sprinkle with 1/4 teaspoon each lemon zest and chopped fennel fronds. Alternatively, transfer 3/4 cup bean mixture to a small skillet before adjusting seasoning in step 2; add one canned, drained, oil-packed wild Pacific sardine, cook while stirring over medium-high heat until the sardine is fully heated and broken into bite-size pieces, then sprinkle with 1/4 teaspoon each lemon zest and fennel fronds.

Full recipe: Heat 8 (3/4-ounce) fully cooked poultry Italian meatballs according to package directions, cut into 3 slices each, nestle on top of each of the servings, and sprinkle with 1 teaspoon each lemon zest and chopped fennel fronds. Alternatively, before adjusting seasoning in step 2, add 4 canned, drained, oil-packed wild Pacific sardines, cook while stirring over medium-high heat until the sardines are fully heated and broken into bite-size pieces, then sprinkle with an additional 1 teaspoon each lemon zest and fennel fronds.

without
Exchanges/Food Choices: 1 Starch, 1 Vegetable, 1/2 Fat
140 calories, 25 calories from fat, 3g total fat, 0g saturated fat, 0g trans fat, 0mg cholesterol, 320mg sodium, 570mg potassium, 21g total carbohydrate, 10g dietary fiber, 2g sugars, 8g protein, 140mg phosphorus

with
Exchanges/Food Choices: 1 Starch, 1 Vegetable, 1 Medium-Fat Meat, 1 Fat
240 calories, 90 calories from fat, 10g total fat, 2.5g saturated fat, 0g trans fat, 55mg cholesterol, 600mg sodium, 680mg potassium, 22g total carbohydrate, 10g dietary fiber, 3g sugars, 16g protein, 250mg phosphorus

Asparagus Frittata Wedge

1 large organic egg

6 large organic egg whites or 3/4 cup pasteurized 100% egg whites

3 tablespoons plain unsweetened almond milk or other plant-based milk

1/4 teaspoon + 1/8 teaspoon sea salt, or to taste

1/8 teaspoon ground turmeric

2 teaspoons canola or grapeseed oil

1 medium red or yellow onion, very thinly sliced

6 ounces trimmed fresh asparagus, thinly sliced on the diagonal (1 1/2 cups)

1/4 cup shredded part-skim mozzarella cheese (1 ounce)

When eating more plant-based food, an entrée may not be as high in protein as a meaty main dish. This frittata is ideally served as a side dish to boost the protein of an entire meal. It's a tasty way to get additional veggies, too.

1. Preheat the oven to 475°F. Whisk together the egg, egg whites, almond milk, 1/4 teaspoon salt, and the turmeric in a medium bowl. Set aside.

2. Heat the oil in a large, ovenproof, nonstick skillet over medium-high heat. Add the onion and sauté until softened, about 5 minutes. Add the asparagus and sauté until the asparagus is al dente, about 5 minutes. Reduce heat to medium-low.

3. Evenly pour in the egg mixture and cook, gently lifting the edges with a spatula to allow the uncooked eggs to run underneath the cooked portion. When the frittata is firm on the bottom and no excess runniness remains on top, about 2 minutes, sprinkle with the cheese.

4. Place the skillet in the oven on the top rack and bake until puffy, about 9 minutes. Remove and let stand for 5 minutes. Sprinkle with the remaining 1/8 teaspoon salt and adjust seasoning. Slice into 4 wedges (be careful; the skillet handle is hot), and serve warm.

{ WITH POULTRY, FISH, OR MEAT }

One serving: Sprinkle 1/2 ounce finely diced lean, uncured ham or rosemary ham onto one-quarter of the frittata immediately after removing it from the oven in step 4. Leave that serving free of the added sea salt in that step. Use a smidgen less than the 1/8 teaspoon salt on the other 3 servings.

Full recipe: Stir 2 ounces finely diced lean, uncured ham or rosemary ham into the onion-asparagus mixture immediately before adding the eggs at the beginning of step 3. Do not add the 1/8 teaspoon salt in step 4.

without

Exchanges/Food Choices: 1 Vegetable, 1 Lean Meat, 1/2 Fat
100 calories, 45 calories from fat, 5g total fat, 1.5g saturated fat, 0g trans fat, 50mg cholesterol, 380mg sodium, 230mg potassium, 5g total carbohydrate, 1g dietary fiber, 2g sugars, 10g protein, 90mg phosphorus

with

Exchanges/Food Choices: 1 Vegetable, 1 Lean Meat, 1 Fat
120 calories, 50 calories from fat, 6g total fat, 1.5g saturated fat, 0g trans fat, 60mg cholesterol, 470mg sodium, 270mg potassium, 6g total carbohydrate, 1g dietary fiber, 2g sugars, 13g protein, 120mg phosphorus

PRODUCT RECOMMENDATIONS

Below is a selected list of grocery picks to use as a helpful guide when shopping for the best-quality ingredients for The With or Without Meat Cookbook recipes.

A

ALMOND BUTTER
MaraNatha No-Salt-Added Creamy & Roasted Organic Almond Butter

ALMOND MILK
SILK Pure Almond Unsweetened Organic Almondmilk

APPLESAUCE (VARIOUS)
Santa Cruz Organic Apple Sauce

B

BACON
Applegate Organics Hickory-Smoked Uncured Sunday Bacon

Applegate Organics Uncured Turkey Bacon

Organic Prairie Organic Hardwood-Smoked Uncured Turkey Bacon

Organic Prairie Organic Uncured Canadian Bacon Slices

BAKED BEANS
Amy's Organic Vegetarian Baked Beans in Tomato Sauce

BEANS (VARIOUS)
Eden Organic No-Salt-Added Beans
Westbrae Natural Organic Beans

BREAD
Bread Alone Whole-Wheat
Sourdough Bread
Food for Life Organic Ezekiel 4:9
Low Sodium Sprouted Whole Grain
Bread

BROTH
Imagine Organic Low Sodium
Vegetable Broth

BUTTER
Horizon Organic Unsalted Butter

C

CHEESE (VARIOUS)
Horizon Organic Shreds
Organic Valley Cheese
Organic Creamery Organic Goat Cheese

CHEESE (VEGAN)
Follow Your Heart Vegan Gourmet
Cheese Alternative

CHICKEN (BREADED)
Applegate Naturals Chicken Patties
Applegate Organics Organic Chicken
Strips
Ian's Organic Chicken Nuggets

CHICKEN (FRESH)
Bell & Evans Air-Chilled Organic
Chicken
Coleman Organic Chicken

CHICKEN (MEATLESS/BREADED)
Gardein Seven Grain Crispy Tenders

COCONUT MILK
Native Forest Unsweetened Organic
Light Coconut Milk

COCONUT MILK BEVERAGE
SILK Pure Coconut Unsweetened
Coconutmilk
So Delicious Dairy Free Unsweetened
Coconut Milk Beverage

COUSCOUS
Rice-Select Organic Whole-Wheat
Couscous

CRISPBREAD
Wasa Light Rye Crispbread

D

DELI MEAT (VARIOUS)
Applegate Deli Meat

DUMPLING WRAPPERS
Tang's Natural Whole-Wheat
Dumpling Wrappers

E

EDAMAME
Seapoint Farms Organic Shelled
Edamame

EGG WHITES
Horizon Organic Pasteurized 100%
Organic Egg Whites
Organic Valley Pasteurized 100%
Organic Egg Whites

ENGLISH MUFFINS
Rudi's Organic Whole-Grain Wheat
English Muffins

H

HEMP SEEDS
Manitoba Harvest Hemp Hearts

HOISIN SAUCE
Steel's Natural Agave Hoisin Sauce

K

KETCHUP
Annie's Naturals Organic Ketchup
Sir Kensington's Classic Ketchup

M

MAYONNAISE
Earth Balance Organic MindfulMayo
Sir Kensington's Classic Mayonnaise

MEATBALLS
Aidells All Natural Italian Style
Chicken Meatballs

N

NEUFCHATEL
Organic Valley Organic Neufchatel
Cheese

NOODLES
Annie Chun's Pad Thai Brown Rice
Noodles
Eden Selected 100% Buckwheat Soba
Noodles
House Foods Tofu Shirataki
Nasoya Pasta Zero Shirataki

O

OIL
Spectrum Cooking Oils

P

PANKO
Ian's Whole-Wheat Panko
Breadcrumbs

PASTA
Barilla Whole Grain Pasta

PEANUT BUTTER
Arrowhead Mills No-Salt-Added
Organic Creamy Peanut Butter
Earth Balance Creamy Natural Peanut
Butter with Flaxseed

PESTO
Academia Barilla Pesto Alla Genovese

PROSCIUTTO AND SPECK
Applegate Naturals Prosciutto
La Quercia Artisan Crafted Sliced Meats

Q

QUARK
Vermont Butter & Cheese Creamery
Quark

R

ROLLS/BUNS
Rudi's Organic 100% Whole-Wheat
Hamburger Buns
Rudi's Organic Wheat Hot Dog Rolls

S

SALAD GREENS (VARIOUS)
Earthbound Farm Organic Salads and
Greens

SALSA
Field Day Organic Medium Salsa
Herdez Salsa Verde

SANDWICH ROUNDS/THINS
Rudi's Organic 100% Whole-Wheat
Sandwich Flatz

SARDINES
Wild Planet Wild Sardines in Extra-Virgin Olive Oil

SAUSAGE (POULTRY)
Applegate Organic Andouille Chicken & Turkey Sausage
Applegate Organic Sweet Italian Chicken & Turkey Sausage

SAUSAGE (VEGAN)
Gardein Breakfast "Sausage" Patties

SMOKED SALMON
St. James Smokehouse Scotch Reserve Scottish Smoked Salmon

T

TAHINI
Arrowhead Mills Organic Sesame Tahini

TEA (GREEN)
Numi Organic Jasmine Green Tea
Stash Organic Premium Green Tea

TOFU (VARIOUS)
Nasoya Organic Extra Firm Tofu
SoyBoy Smoked Tofu
Twin Oaks "More than Tofu" Ready-to Eat Tofus
Wildwood SproutTofu Organic Savory Baked Tofu

TOMATO PRODUCTS (VARIOUS)
Eden Organic Tomato Products (in amber glass jars)
Muir Glen Organic Fire Roasted Crushed Tomatoes

TORTILLA CHIPS
Food Should Taste Good Blue Corn Tortilla Chips
Garden of Eatin' Corn Tortilla Chips

TORTILLAS (VARIOUS)
Food for Life Ezekiel 4:9 Sprouted Grain Tortillas
Food for Life Sprouted Corn Tortillas
Rudi's Organic Whole-grain Tortillas

TUNA
Wild Planet Wild Albacore Tuna

V

VEGETABLES (FROZEN)
Birds Eye Pure & Simple Frozen Vegetables
Cascadian Farm Organic Premium Bagged Frozen Vegetables

W

WHOLE GRAINS (VARIOUS)
Arrowhead Mills Grains
Bob's Red Mill Grains

WONTON WRAPPERS
Tang's Natural Whole-Wheat Wonton Wrapper

WORCESTERSHIRE SAUCE (VEGAN)
Annie's Naturals Organic Worcestershire Sauce

Y

YOGURT
Chobani Plain Non-Fat Greek Yogurt
Stonyfield Plain Organic Non-Fat Greek Yogurt
Stonyfield Plain Organic Non-Fat Yogurt

INDEX

V

Y

Z